Longevity Training-Book 5-Having Love in Your Heart

This book is a transcription and reproduction of the training course materials from Course #5 "Having Love in Your Heart".

It is all about Unconditional Love—which is a real force-not just an abstract thought process.

You can learn to open your heart chakra through exercises provided in this book and other "Heart Rose" meditation exercises.

Having a real open heart experience will help build your connection to others and strengthen your immune system.

Learning to experience Unconditional Love will be a major experience in your life and help you in many ways you can't think of right now.

Longevity Training-Book 5-Having Love in Your Heart

Longevity Training-Book 5-Having Love in Your Heart

Copyright Page

The book is copyrighted for 2018

Longevity Training-Book 5-Having Love in Your Heart

By Martin K. Ettington

ISBN: 9781791768751

Printed in the United States of America

Longevity Training-Book 5-Having Love in Your Heart

Longevity Training-Book 5-Having Love in Your Heart

Other books by Martin K. Ettington

Longevity Training-Book 5-Having Love in Your Heart

Strange and Ancient Places in the USA
A Theory of Ancient Prehistory And
        Giant Aliens
<u>Aliens and Space</u>
Aliens and Secret Technology
Aliens Are Already Among Us
Designing and Building Space Colonies
Humanity and the Universe

All About Moon Bases
All About Mars Journeys and Settlement
The Space and Aliens Six Books Bundle
A Theory of Ancient Prehistory and
        Giant Aliens
The Space Colonies and Space
        Structures Coloring Book
All About Asteroids

<u>The Longevity Training Series</u>

(A transcription of the online Multimedia Longevity Coaching Training Program)

The Personal Longevity Training Series-Book1-Long Lived Persons
The Personal Longevity Training Series-Book2-Your Soul's Purpose
The Personal Longevity Training Series-Book3-Enable Your Life Urge
The Personal Longevity Training Series-Book4-Your Spiritual Connection
The Personal Longevity Training Series-Book5-Having Love in Your Heart
The Personal Longevity Training Series-Book6-Energy Body Health
The Personal Longevity Training Series-Book7-The Science of Longevity
The Personal Longevity Training Series-Book8-Physical Body Health
The Personal Longevity Training Series-Book9-Avoiding Accidents
The Personal Longevity Training Series-Book10-Implementing These Principles

The Personal Longevity Training Series-Books One Thru Ten

These books are all available in digital and printed formats from my
website and on Amazon, Barnes & Noble, Apple ITunes, and many other sites

My Books Website is: http://mkettingtonbooks.com

Longevity Training-Book 5-Having Love in Your Heart

<u>Signup for our Mailing List to get the following:</u>

1) A discount coupon for 25% discount on all books on our site

2) Occasional Notices of new books available

3) Occasional Email on other offerings of ours (Monthly)

Go to this link to sign-up:

http://personal-longevity.com/mkebooks/emailsignup/

And click this link to get the FREE 102 page Ebook titled "Secrets of Many Things"

If you have any questions about this book or other subjects please contact the Author at:

mke@mkettingtonbooks.com

Longevity Training-Book 5-Having Love in Your Heart

Longevity Training-Book 5-Having Love in Your Heart

Table of Contents

Introduction..1
PLP Concepts Overview 11
Course #5 Intro Video..15
Learning About an Open Heart 19
Chapter 1: Introduction 19
Chapter 2: The History of Love 22
Chapter 3: Love and Affection..........................32
Chapter 4: Love and Friendship.......................35
Chapter 5: Love and Romance 39
Chapter 6: Love Defined Through Quotes 43
Chapter 7: Unconditional LOVE........................50
Chapter 8: The Story of Ram Dass 53
Chapter 9: Paths to Unconditional Love 55
Chapter 10: Exercises in Unconditional Love ...59
Chapter 11: Loving in the Now..........................63
Imagine the Greatest Love in Your Life 67
Chapter 12: Summary of Love from the Heart...69
Our Illusions 71
Chapter 2: Lack of Happiness is due to illusions...........71
Chapter 6: The Ego makes true happiness impossible.74
....74
Chapter 16: Limited Lifespan is an Illusion 77
a.   Long Lived Persons 77
b.   Breaking the Habit of Dying 80
Chapter 17: The Reality Illusion........................82
a.   Metaphysics on Reality.................................83
b.   Modern Science on Reality...........................84
The Heart Rose Exercise 87
Gratitude Now..91
Foreword..91
Gratitude Now 91

Chapter 2: Don't Resist 96
Chapter 3: Be Satisfied 99
Chapter 4: Forgive 102
Chapter 5: Give...105
The Power of Gratitude 109
Summary 129

Longevity Training-Book 5-Having Love in Your Heart

Introduction

Back in 2008 I became very interested in the field of Longevity and Physical Immortality. After a lot of research this led me to my first book on the subject "Physical Immortality: A History and How to Guide". This book was pretty popular and I wanted to continue learning about Longevity and what things we could do about it in our lives.

The subject continued to fascinate me to the point that I developed a Longevity Coaching program over a couple of years starting in 2011. This online training program was multimedia—consisting of videos, my writings on longevity to read, online exercises, and tests for each of ten courses. It also included a lot of additional resources for each course including extra courses on how to become a successful Longevity Coach. A student who completed the training and tests successfully would become certified as a "Longevity Coach" and authorized to teach this material to others.

I developed a set of ten principles on longevity which are as follows:

The 10 Principles of Personal Longevity are:

- The Reality of Long Lived People
- Defining Your Purpose in Life
- Enabling the Life Urge
- Your Spiritual Health
- Having Love in Your Heart
- Energy Body Health
- The Science of Longevity
- Physical Body Health
- Using your Intuition for Safety
- Implementation of these principles

What are the 10 Principles all about?

The Reality of Long Lived People

The first principle is where I provide lots of evidence of people who have lived well over the age of 120 years old to 150-180-200, and even a 256 year old man from China:

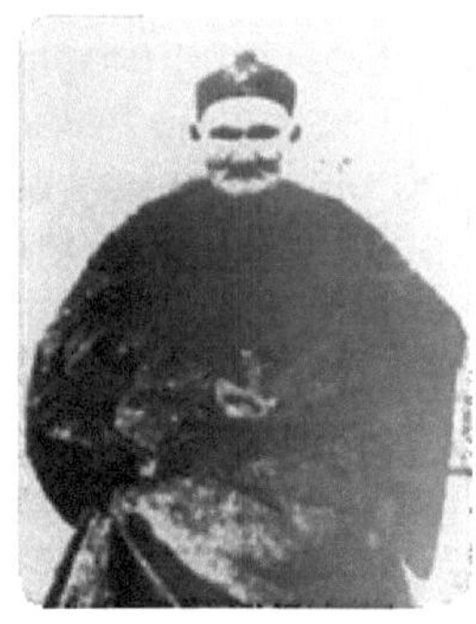

LI CHING-YUN: The Longest Lived person of record-256 Years (Source-The New York Times-May 6, 1933)

The Second Principle of Life Purpose

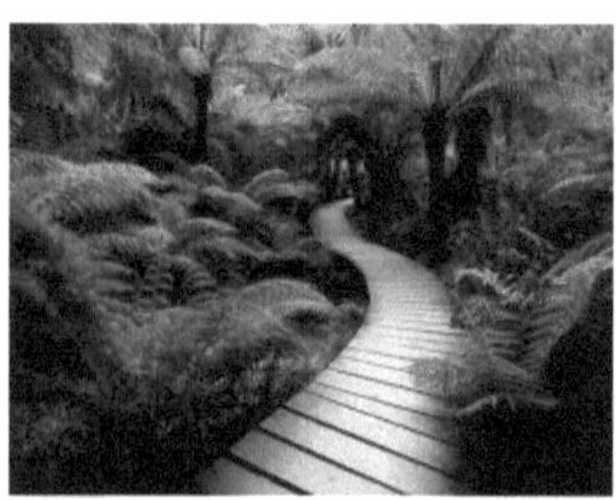

One of the things that occurred to me when I was putting the 10 principles together was that if one doesn't have a reason to live, or purpose in life--then what is the point?

This meant I had to add a very important step of how you can develop your own life purpose, or bring it up to date with your phase in life. Without reviewing your purpose-- then none of the rest of the principles matter.

Enabling the Life Urge

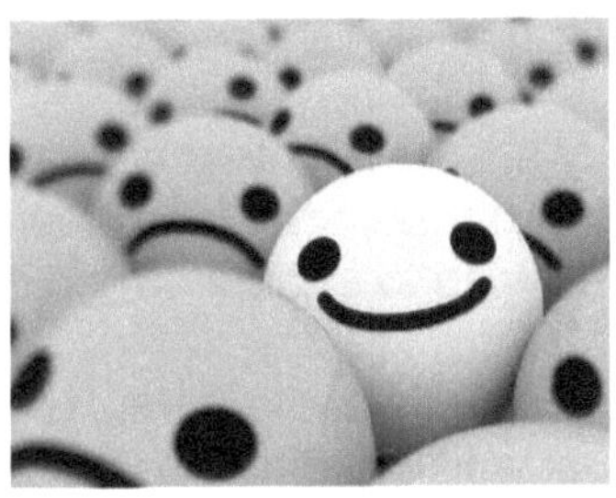

Have you ever realized how we are all programmed to expect to live through certain stages in life and then die? It's so common in our society that we don't think it odd that we expect to die at a certain age?

Have you ever heard radio ads saying "You are getting up in your sixties and seventies" so it's time to come out to our cemetery and buy a plot"

How ridiculous is this? And do you see how much our subconscious has been programmed towards death?

This principle is all about reprogramming ourselves to have a more positive outlook on life and its possibilities.

Having a Spiritual Connection in Your Life

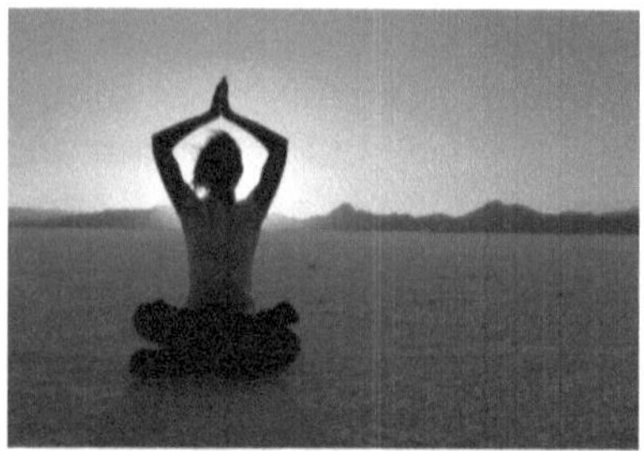

Most of us innately understand that we have a spiritual core in the center of our being. It is this spiritual core that we need to connect with to enable our physical health too.

It doesn't matter what religion you are. Regular meditation, deep prayer, or just walking in the woods helps you make and keep that connection in your life.

Having Love in Your Heart

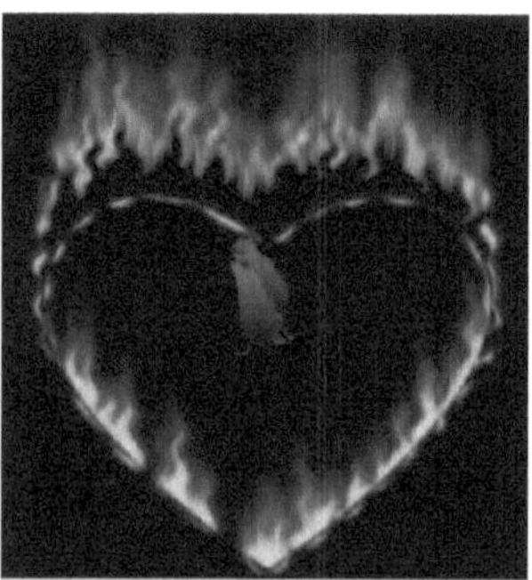

One of the most important things I learned in the last five years was that Unconditional Love is a real and physical thing. It is a powerful energy force in life and not just a philosophical belief system.

I considered it so important that I added it as a separate principle of longevity.

True Unconditional Love is healing, embodies happiness, and is a powerful part of our vital forces.

Energy Body Health

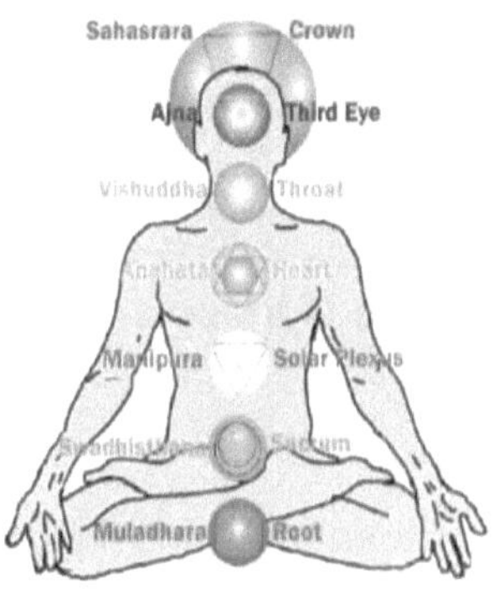

We all have an energy body which is part of our vital forces. The Indians talk about the "Chakras" and the Chinese talk about "Energy Meridians" in Acupuncture.

We should all learn different practices to keep our vital forces flowing for maximum health and vitality.

The Science of Longevity

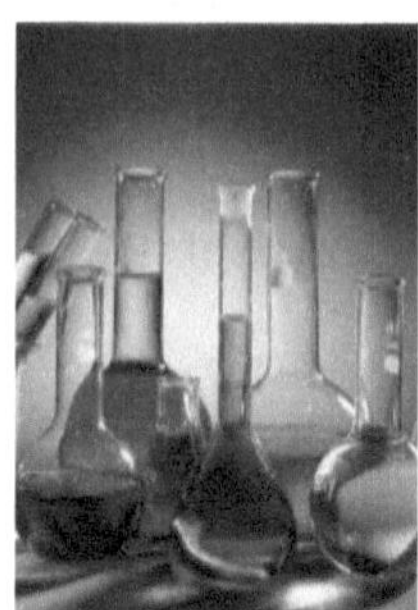

Science and Medicine are making new discoveries all the time that we can take advantage of to extend our lives. Why not take advantage of these discoveries which provide new therapies and supplements to increase our longevity.

There is also a lot we can learn from plants and animals. We all share the same genetic basis.

Some of these plants and animals live thousands of years and some cells are immortal.

What can we learn from them to apply to our lives?

Physical Body Health

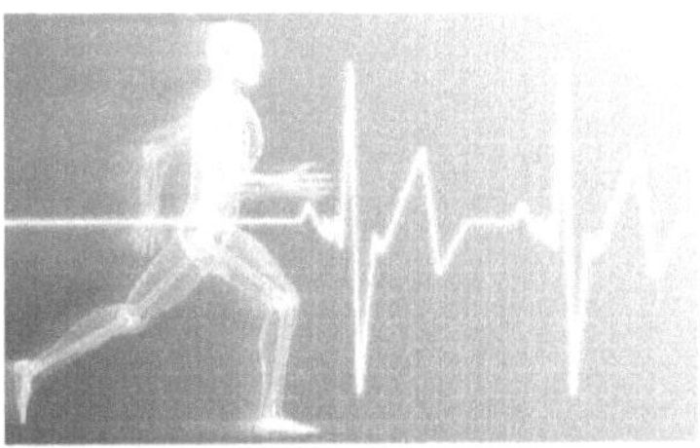

There are many types of supplements used for anti-aging for thousands of years. What can we learn about them that we can apply to our lives?

What other considerations about our physical health does nontraditional or alternative medicine offer?

Using Your Intuition for Safety

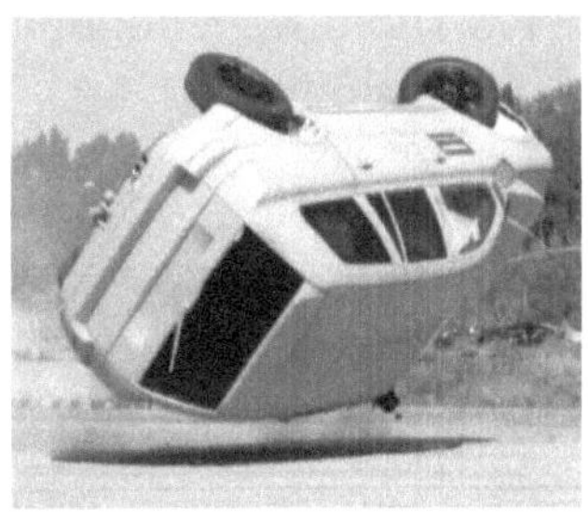

Once you have established your own long term health then what is the greatest danger you face?

ACCIDENTS

We can learn to use our intuition to make us safer as well as see potential future events which may be good too.

Why not open up to the possibilities of how our spirit has this natural ability in all of us?

Implementing These Principles in Your Life

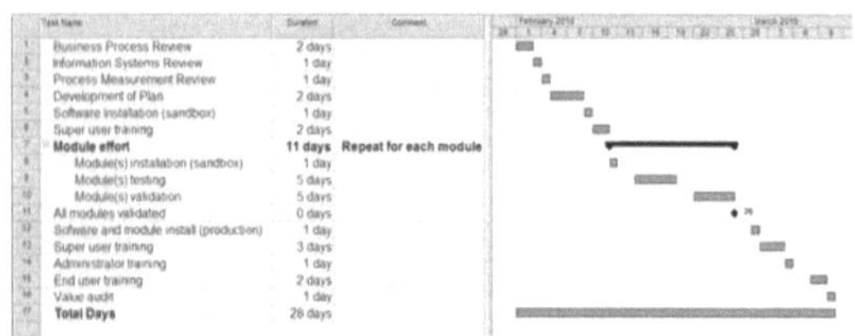

It's nice to read about all these concepts, but how can you really apply them to your own life?

This is what the chapter on implementation is all about, and it helps you plan a lifelong change in your health focus to live these principles and truly experience long term health, greater happiness, and extended longevity.

For five years I amended and improved these materials which now include a lot more information and helpful concepts for students wanting to improve their longevity and those of others.

I transcribed my videos and other materials to this book so you can read it all, and later hear it in an AudioBook.

This book is priced pretty inexpensively, compared to the online training and certification program which sells in total for $1,995 USD. If you are interested in taking the entire online program at a major discount, then please contact me at:

Marty@personal-longevity.com

Hope you enjoy these materials since when applied correctly they will significantly change your life.

PLP Concepts Overview

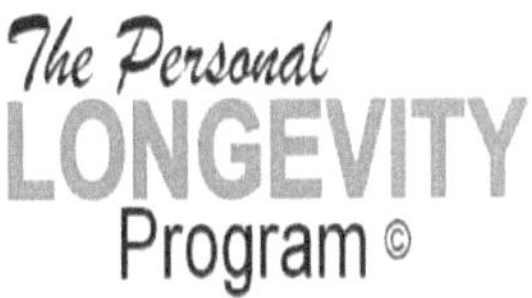

(Transcription of overview video)

Hello I'm Martin Ettington and I'd like to introduce you to the Personal Longevity Program which is an integrated holistic approach to long-term health. In this video we will only cover the high level concepts which comprise individual courses in the coaching certificate program for personal longevity.

The first concept is that long lived people exist and have existed for hundreds of thousands of years. We cover in the first course all about their records; along with people not only in places you might think like India, but in Europe and the United States-people who've lived long lives and well documented cases.

We discuss people who have lived well over the age of 120 and even the case of a Chinaman who lived to 256 years old. Plus a lot of mythology about people who have lived even longer lives so you get an idea that extending your life much longer than we think is currently medically and scientifically possible is certainly something that can happen.

The second course's concept has to do with finding your souls purpose. The point of wanting to live a long life is to know what your purpose in life is, so we go through some readings and some exercises to help you determine where soul's purpose in life is. Then doing goals as a fundamental concept so you will know the motivations in your life.

Third is the "Psychology of Living" also known by certain practitioners as "Removing the death Urge". The psychology of living has to do with seeking a positive image about your ability to live a long time. We tend to be programmed from birth about the idea that we are going to go through certain stages in our life as a child, as a teenager, and as adults. It's about reprogramming your subconscious as to the possibilities of a long life.

I've also learned in my life that it is very important to be able open your heart to unconditional love. When you're able to love unconditionally it also helps increase the strength of your immune system and fight off disease. So this is an aspect of spiritual growth. The courses also cover unconditional love and energy body forces. Managing your energy body is an important component of who you are in having energy working properly in your body and is another aspect of health for the length of longevity.

There are many types of scientific and medical research which are being done today and which will contribute to human longevity in the future.

Do you know that the average lifespan in the United States in 1900 was only about 40 years? We have doubled lifespan in the last century with current technologies but things under way in terms of scientific and medical improvements will help extend your lives further.

Also in this course on longevity we will cover a lot of the concepts which are being researched by scientists today. There are suggestions for more things you can do to do to use this science to improve your health along with physical supplements.

A unique thing that I thought about and decided to offer in these courses has to do with all my experiences in prophecy and how I was able to change outcomes on accidents that would occur to me by using simple exercises you can learn to change these outcomes. If you're in great health often the biggest thing you have to worry about are accidents.

We also provide guidelines you can follow on a daily basis and plans you can make to live healthier and happier and have a much longer life than you ever thought possible.

Thank you for listening !

Course #5 Intro Video

(Transcription of Video)

Hello this is Marty Ettington I'd like to welcome you to course number Five-"Having Love In Your Heart". This is part of the ten course sequence of the personal longevity coaching program.

You might wonder why would I put a course like this on the health and longevity program. And the reason is that it's an important aspect of spirituality, happiness, and health. I've been blessed to have this experience in my life and I want to share it with you and also provide you more information and some exercises. So if you don't already have an open heart you can learn how to do it yourself. I've found it invaluable in my life through many of my experiences.

I believe that having a real open heart is an important aspect of spirituality and long-term health. It gives you a new dimension of happiness-kind of another dimension in terms of the way you relate to people. It helps improve your immune system and I even had a friend of mine recently tell me how doing exercises on energizing and opening his heart-actually helped him clear some artery blockages. I'm not going to claim it will do this for you, but he found it had some real physical health benefits.

Historically there's been four types of love that I think were best defined by C.S. Lewis in the book "The Four Loves". The first love he talked about is Empathy-using the Greek terms was "Storge" which has to do with affection. The affection that you feel for friends and other people in your life. Also it could be for children or parents.

Then there's "Philia" which is friendship. Friendship of many different types-more of a distance type of love but still important.

"Eros" is probably the best-known type of love which is talking about romance and physical intimacy between people and what you find in marriage and other intimate relationships.

But probably the most under realized and least understood form of love is "Agape" or "Unconditional Love" where we might think we understand it through our philosophical approach. And the things which were taught and in religion but it's actually something you can experience physically which is very intense. And I'll try and describe what it feels like.

I had my first experiences of unconditional love-when I learned this Heart Rose exercise or visualization exercise I went through a few years ago. And I had these intense feelings of energy and a very powerful experience of love for everybody around me and everything around me. It was like coming out of me-not something that I was drawing on. It was a really incredible feeling and then later on my heart opened on a regular basis and it was like it filled a hole that had been there for most of my life.

A hole that I tried to fill through relationships and it was never really filled until my heart opened. And this actual energy came in and filled me-empowered me, and made me-I think a more whole person. So there seem to be several paths to unconditional love. Some of them can just be over a period of time through leading a spiritual religious life and thinking more about God flowing through you. But there's some more powerful techniques also that can work in the shorter term that involves gratitude and thanking exercises from your heart. These are taught by Dr. Demartini and some books I'm going to have here in the course about gratitude and thanking. And then there's some different visualization exercises you can do later in the course. You'll see one called the "Heart Rose" visualization which is a great exercise to do and also gave me a lot of great experiences.

So I hope you enjoy this and get a lot out of it and don't forget to do the test at the end of the course which is important for your certification in the personal longevity program. Thank you very much.

Learning About an Open Heart

Chapter 1: Introduction

> *Everything that exists is both hunter and prey.*
> *What is it that we hunt? Humans hunt for love.*
> *We feel that we need that love, because we believe*
> *we don't have love,*
> *because we don't love ourselves.*
> *We hunt for love in other humans just like us,*
> *expecting to get love from them when these*
> *humans are in the condition as we are.*
> *We are hunting for love, when the love we need is*
> *inside ourselves.*
> *-Don Miguel Ruiz*

We all know something about love because the reality permeates our daily lives.

But something is missing in our daily lives—and we don't know why.

We may feel that we don't have enough love:

- That we are not loved
- That we are not worthy of being loved (1)
- That someone who loved us no longer feels the same
- That love within our own families may not be the same that it used to be
- That other people are loved more than us.

Or we may feel very happy sometimes:

- The happiness of being with our significant other—girlfriend, boyfriend, or spouse

- The love we have as parents for children
- The love for pets
- The spiritual love for total strangers
- The love for a city, state, country, or humanity in general

In any event, the feelings of love go silent—why can't we always be happy with love?

To get a better handle on how love affects our lives, we should also understand the different types of love we experience.

C.S. Lewis wrote one of the definitive classics on love titled "The Four Loves"; covering the subject of Love and he defined that four types of Love exist.

The types of Love C.S. Lewis defines in Greek with their English words are:

Storge-Affection

What people feel for family members and others who may be together by chance. It is the most natural and widely diffused of the loves.

Philia-Friendship

This is love between friends. Friendship is a strong bond existing between persons who share common interests or activities. It's the least biological, organic, instinctive, and necessary of the four Loves.

Eros-Romance

Eros is about being in Love or loving another. This is separate from sexuality although the two are often related.

Agape-Unconditional Love

Agape is the most unconditional love which can happen no matter what the circumstance. It is often stressed as a Christian virtue although agape is not specific to any religion and can be experienced by anyone.

****

My objective in this book is to cover the history of love, the different types of love, and how we can learn to live in the highest form of love—which we call "unconditional love".

Unconditional Love is a very spiritual state and most of us experience it rarely in our lives-if at all.

If you can improve the force of love acting in your life and get an uplifted attitude from reading this book—then I will have accomplished my goal.

Chapter 2: The History of Love

Why look at Love in History? I think the history of any subject can help us understand where we have been as a civilization, and where we may want to go into the future….

One good way to look at the history of love is to recount some of the most famous love stories in history:

How about the story of Romeo & Juliet by William Shakespeare: (Amo Life, 2012)

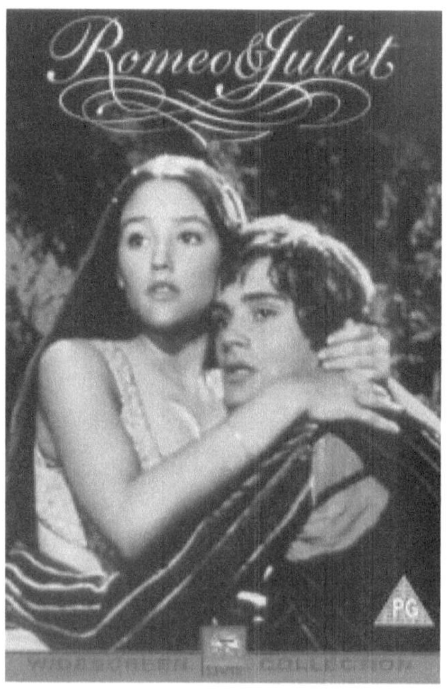

These are probably the most famous lovers ever-even though fictional. This couple has become a synonym for love itself. Romeo and Juliet is a tragedy by William Shakespeare. Their love story is very tragic.

The tale of two teenagers from two feuding families who fall in love at first sight and then marry, become true lovers and then risk it all for their love. To take your own life for your husband or wife is definitely a sign of true love. Their "untimely deaths" ultimately unite their feuding households.

This story of teenage Eros shows the imperfection of love between humans. I'm not condemning it—but is that all there is?

****

What about the oldest love story which may be true?

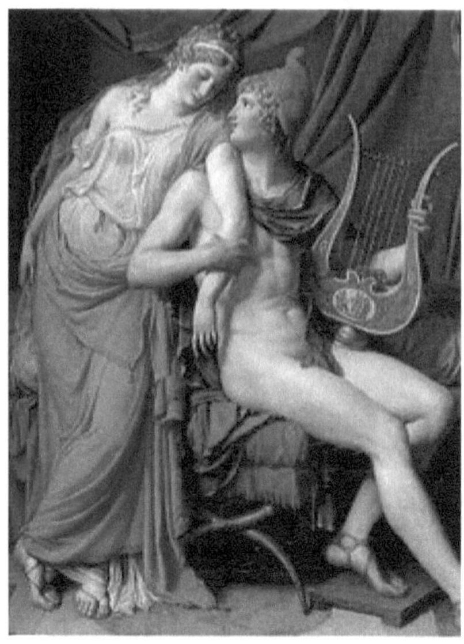

Recounted in Homer's Iliad, the story of Helen of Troy and the Trojan War is a Greek heroic legend, combining fact and fiction. Helen of Troy is considered one the most beautiful women in all literature. She was married to Menelaus, king of Sparta. Paris, son of King Priam of Troy, fell in love with Helen and abducted her, taking her back to Troy. The Greeks assembled a great army, led by Menelaus's brother, Agamemnon, to retrieve Helen. Troy was destroyed. Helen returned safely to Sparta, where she lived happily with Menelaus for the rest of her life.

Was this love or just desire?

****

Anthony and Cleopatra is another very old love story which is supposed to be true:

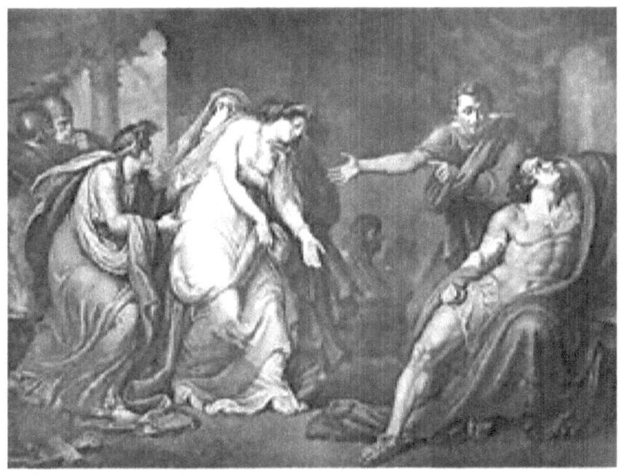

The true love story of Antony and Cleopatra is one of the most memorable, intriguing and moving of all times. The story of these two historical characters had later been dramatized by William Shakespeare and is still staged all over the world.

The relationship of Antony and Cleopatra is a true test of love. They fell in love at first sight. The relationship between these two powerful people put the country of Egypt in a powerful position. But their love affair outraged the Romans who were wary of the growing powers of the Egyptians. Despite all the threats, Anthony and Cleopatra got married.

It is said that while fighting a battle against Romans, Antony got false news of Cleopatra's death. Shattered, he fell on his sword. When Cleopatra learned about Antony's death, she was shocked. And she took her own life. Great love demands great sacrifices.

****

Maybe it's something about Greek culture that they had so many words for love, and that they have some of the oldest stories of love we know:

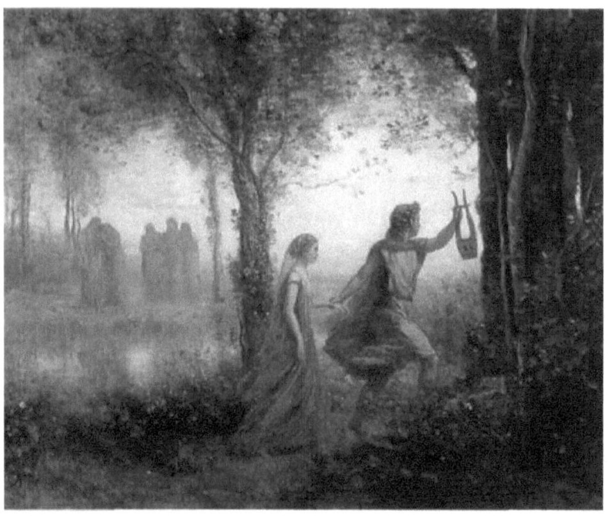

Orpheus and Eurydice story is an ancient Greek tale of desperate love. Orpheus fell deeply in love with and married Eurydice, a beautiful nymph. They were very much in love and very happy together. Aristaeus, a Greek god of the land and agriculture, became quite fond of Eurydice, and actively pursued her. While fleeing from Aristaeus, Eurydice ran into a nest of snakes which bit her fatally on her legs.

Distraught, Orpheus played such sad songs and sang so mournfully that all the nymphs and gods wept. On their advice, Orpheus traveled to the underworld and by his music softened the hearts of Hades and Persephone (he was the only person ever to do so), who agreed to allow Eurydice to return with him to earth on one condition: he should walk in front of her and not look back until they both had reached the upper world. In his anxiety he forgot that both needed to be in the upper world, and he turned to look at her, and she vanished for the second time, but now forever.

****

In more modern times, Napoleon and Josephine had quite a story to tell:

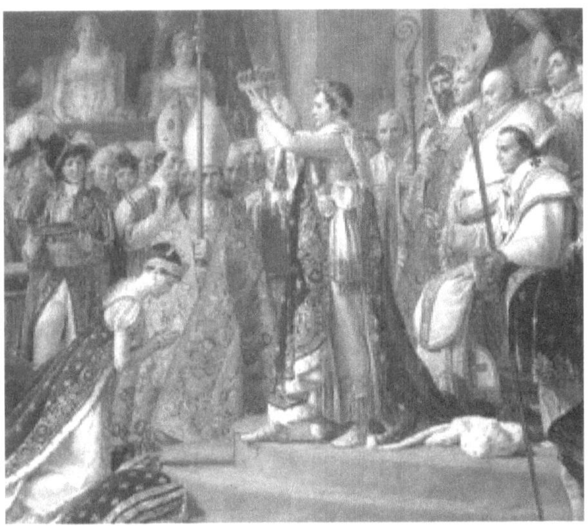

A marriage of convenience, at age 26 Napoleon took a fancy to Josephine--An older, prominent, and most importantly wealthy woman. As time drew on, Napoleon fell deeply in love with Josephine, and she with him, but that didn't deter the adultery on both sides-their mutual respect for one another kept them together, and their burning passion between them didn't falter, and was genuine.

They eventually split, as Napoleon deeply required something Josephine could not give him, an heir. Sadly they parted ways, both bearing the love and passion in their hearts, for all eternity.

****

Historical accounts of love are mainly about Eros and offer some glimpses of Unconditional Love, but don't really give us any guidance as to how to find it.

Love in the Bible (Various, The Holy Bible)

The Holy Bible is the core teaching of Christianity and stresses Love for spiritual growth and happiness in one's life.

Jesus taught about loving God in many different ways and the Old and New Testaments provide many of the most famous quotes on love.

Several quotes illustrate the themes of love in the Bible including unconditional love which we will focus on later in this book.

Probably the most famous quote on love in the Bible is used today in many weddings and refers to what we call unconditional love:

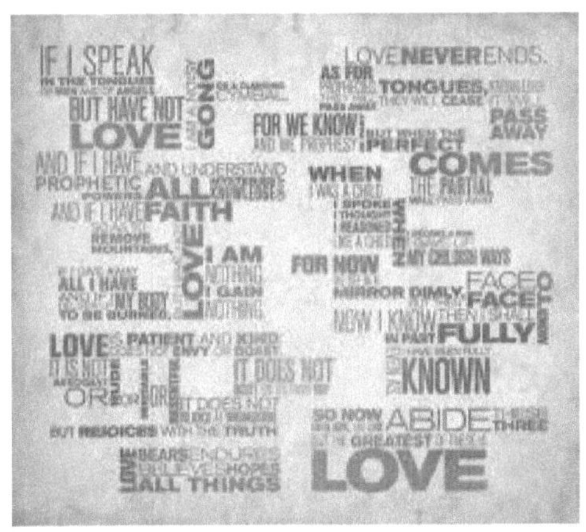

1 Corinthians 13:4-13 *Love is patient and kind; love does not envy or boast; it is not arrogant or rude. It does not insist on its own way; it is not irritable or resentful-it does not rejoice at*

> **wrongdoing, but rejoices with the truth. Love bears all things, believes all things, hopes all things, endures all things. Love never ends**. *As for prophecies, they will pass away; as for tongues, they will cease; as for knowledge, it will pass away. For we know in part and we prophesy in part, but when the perfect comes, the partial will pass away. When I was a child, I spoke like a child, I thought like a child, I reasoned like a child. When I became a man, I gave up childish ways. For now we see in a mirror dimly, but then face to face. Now I know in part; then I shall know fully, even as I have been fully known. So now faith, hope, and love abide, these three; but the greatest of these is love.*

Another quote on loving your enemies implies a spiritual and unattached love which is above the "normal" types of love:

> LUKE 6:35
> But love your enemies, do good to them, and lend to them without expecting to get anything back. Then your reward will be great, and you will be sons of the Most High, because he is kind to the ungrateful and wicked.

Love has the benefit of overcoming fear:

> 1 JOHN 4:18-19
> There is no fear in love. But perfect love drives out fear, because fear has to do with punishment. The one who fears is not made perfect in love. We love because he first loved us.

Another way of visualizing unconditional love:

SONG OF SOLOMON 8:4-8 DAUGHTERS OF JERUSALEM, I CHARGE YOU: DO NOT AROUSE OR AWAKEN LOVE UNTIL IT SO DESIRES. WHO IS THIS COMING UP FROM THE DESERT LEANING ON HER LOVER? UNDER THE APPLE TREE I ROUSED YOU; THERE YOUR MOTHER CONCEIVED YOU, THERE SHE WHO WAS IN LABOR GAVE YOU BIRTH. PLACE ME LIKE A SEAL OVER YOUR HEART, LIKE A SEAL ON YOUR ARM; FOR LOVE IS AS STRONG AS DEATH, ITS JEALOUSY UNYIELDING AS THE GRAVE. IT BURNS LIKE BLAZING FIRE, LIKE A MIGHTY FLAME. MANY WATERS CANNOT QUENCH LOVE; RIVERS CANNOT WASH IT AWAY. IF ONE WERE TO GIVE ALL THE WEALTH OF HIS HOUSE FOR LOVE, IT WOULD BE UTTERLY SCORNED. WE HAVE A YOUNG SISTER, AND HER BREASTS ARE NOT YET GROWN. WHAT SHALL WE DO FOR OUR SISTER FOR THE DAY SHE IS SPOKEN FOR?

How else can we love all our neighbors except with the love of God?

MATTHEW 22:37-39

Jesus replied: "Love the Lord your God with all your heart and with all your soul and with all your mind." This is the first and greatest commandment. And the second is like it: 'Love your neighbor as yourself.'

Chapter 3: Love and Affection

Love begins from birth and can be easily carried out throughout life by the human necessity of affection. People strive and live for lasting affection. It is healthy to feel emotions and feel nurtured. Through these states of feeling, love can be brought forward in a positive manner. So positive in fact that affectionate behavior is linked to many health benefits.

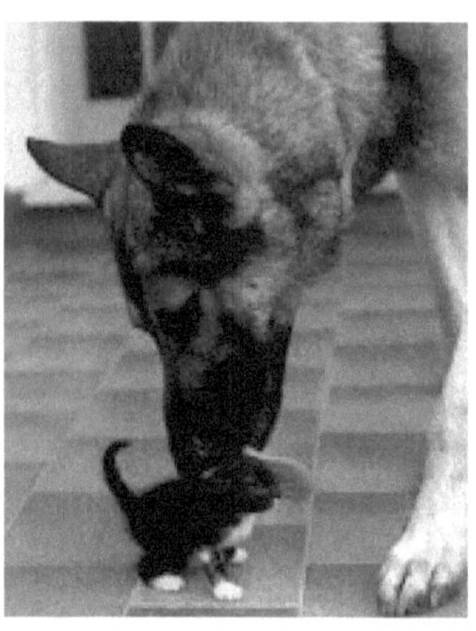

According to psychologist Henry Murray, there are five types of affection needs. These include affiliation, nurturance, play, rejection, and succorance. Examples of these types of affections include the following:

- Spending time with other people
- Taking care of another person
- Having fun with others
- Rejecting other people
- Being helped or protected by others

These affection needs are both on a conscious and unconscious level, just as our love for others can be. Ask yourself if you are participating in the 5 types of affection. What areas may you be lacking in? Acknowledge your truth for you have just discovered what may or may not be missing links to your own pleasantness, pleasure, and displeasure. Once having realized this, you are then able to take charge with how you want to feel with yourself, especially in direct relation to love. Are you experiencing tension or relaxation? Excitement or depression?

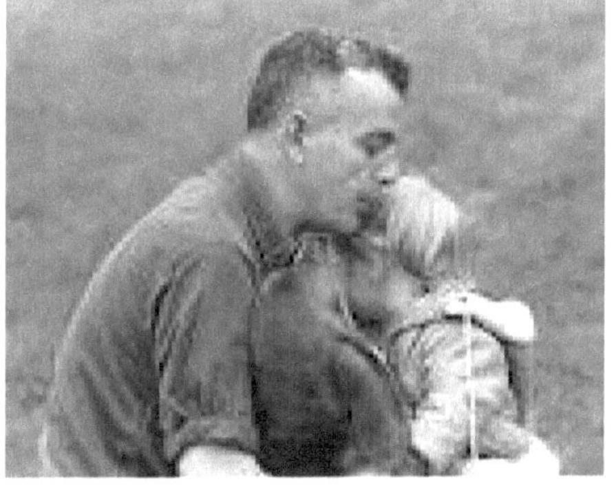

Having answered these questions and digesting your answers, dig deep into the 5 types of affection and fill in those blocks one step at a time. Keep track of the small steps you make toward becoming a well-rounded, affectionate person. Thank yourself and others. Feel gratitude around you. You have the power to feel and express your love. You are love!

Feeling the love today?? Reach out to someone special or perhaps someone you have been wanting to connect with lately.

JM

Chapter 4: Love and Friendship

Without friends, love is nonexistent. Love is eternal and unconditional through the relationship with a strong friend. Friendship can be eternal through knowing someone on such a deep level that forms through trust, listening to one another, and experiencing new ways of life. It is important to find compatibility when choosing our best friends, wisely (!), through the psychological and emotional levels we know as ourselves.

After all, a friendship can many times be summed up to what Aristotle quotes, "What is a friend? A single soul, dwelling in two bodies." A true friend can be formed through one warm heart reaching out to another. Love is found through those feelings of empathy and sympathy that forms the bond between lasting friendships.

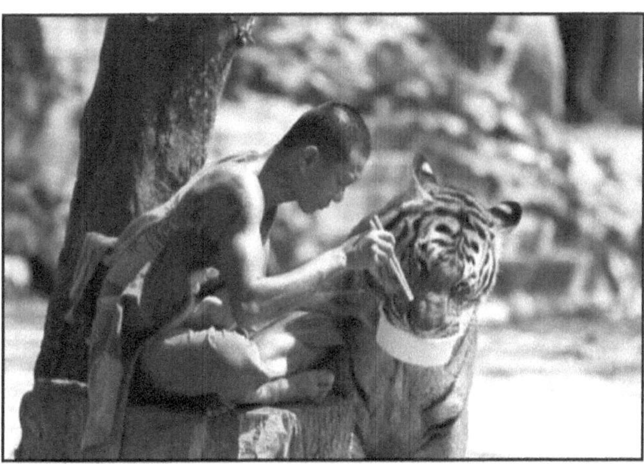

So how can love be formed through friendship? Below is a list of popular answers taken from well-known books and quotes from people:

Friendship is a sweet attraction of the heart, towards the merit we esteem, or the "perfections we admire; and produces a mutual inclination between two persons, to promote each other's interest, knowledge, virtue, and happiness."- Wellins Calott

"Some people come into our lives and quickly go. Some stay for a while and leave footprints on our hearts. And we are never, ever the same." –Unknown

"Friendship involves many things, but above all, the power of going out of one's self and appreciating what is noble and loving in another." –Thomas Hughes

"There is a magnet in your heart that will attract true friends. That magnet is unselfishness, thinking of others first…when you learn to live for others, they will live for you." –Paramahansa Yogananda

"No love, no friendship can cross the path of our destiny without leaving some mark on it forever." –Francois Mauriac

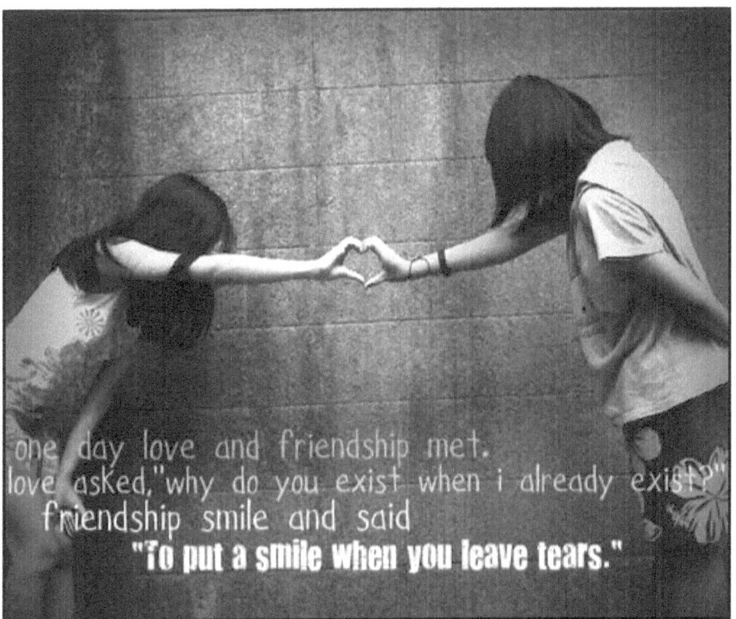

I hope these quotes leave you with a warm heart and you are able to move forward in your friendships with others, and most importantly, your friendship to yourself!

JM

Chapter 5: Love and Romance

We have all experienced love in many forms with different people, animals, and even hobbies. But what about romantic love? Romance is defined by Webster as "A love affair."

An emotional involvement takes place between two people and their time can be shared with one another in enthusiasm, mystery, pleasure and fascination. If these feelings are formed and bonded between the two, a spiritual relationship may also unfold into a romantic relationship filled with even more love and meaning.

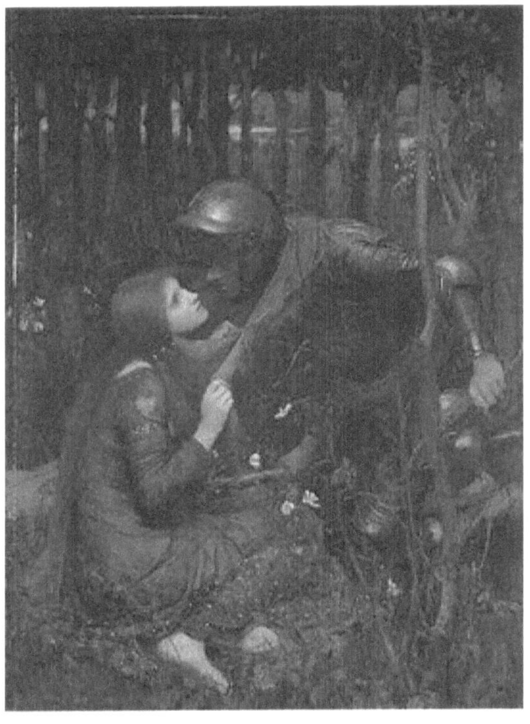

"People compose poetry, novels, sitcoms for love," says Helen Fisher, anthropologist at Rutgers University. "They live for love, die for love, kill for love. It can be stronger than the drive to stay alive."

Listed below are some of the key factors for a successful romantic relationship:

- Tell your partner you love them
- Be there for your partner
- Show affection and share yourself
- Give gifts to show you care
- Allow "alone time" for yourself
- Take no-thing for granted

What are some of the things you have done for others that affected them in a positive way? Think about your strength as a person and how you can utilize your gifts to others.'

"You don't love someone for their looks, or their clothes, or for their fancy car, but because they sing a song only you can hear."

To the beauty of romance,

JM

Chapter 6: Love Defined Through Quotes

Sometimes one of the best ways to understand Love is to contemplate quotes by famous people on the subject. Here are some of our favorites to meditate on…

10 Quotes on Love
Here are some wonderful words put together from a few brilliant minds. Along with the quotes are some pictures to feel the soul. Enjoy <3
(NAD does not claim rights to any of the pictures posted.)

"Love is the beauty of the soul." St. Aurelius Augustine

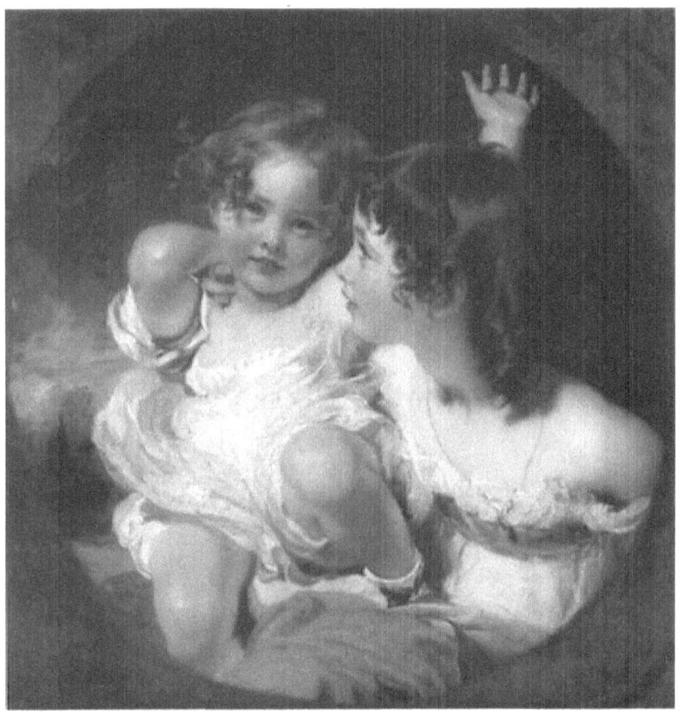

"If the sight of the blue skies fills you with joy, if a blade of grass springing up in the fields has power to move you, if the simple things of nature have a message that you understand, rejoice, for your soul is alive…"
Eleonora Duse

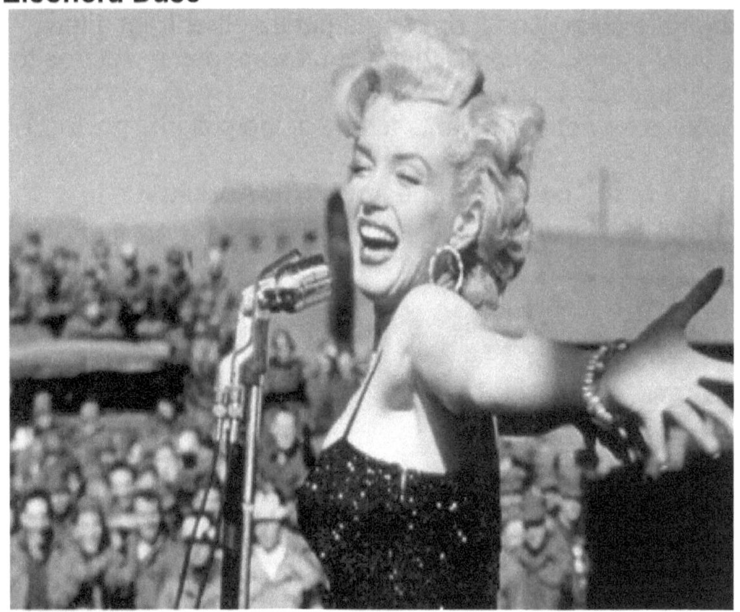

"Harmony is pure love, for love is a concerto." Lope de Vega

"The best and most beautiful things in the world cannot be seen or even touched. They must be felt with the heart."
Helen Keller

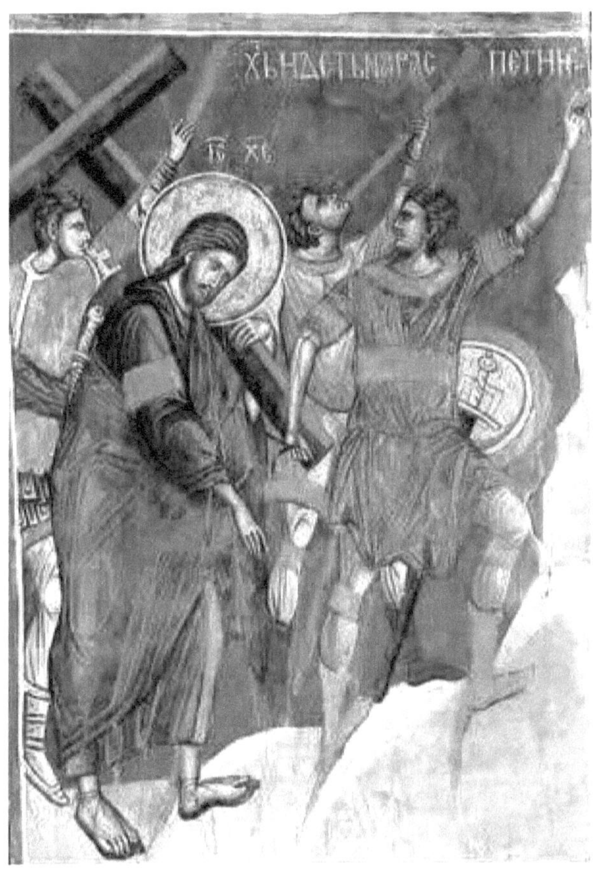

"There is only one happiness in life, to love and be loved."
George Sand

"And, when he shall die, take him and cut him out in little
stars, and he will make the face of Heaven so fine that all
the world will be in love with night and pay no worship to
the garish sun." {Romeo and Juliet} – William Shakespeare

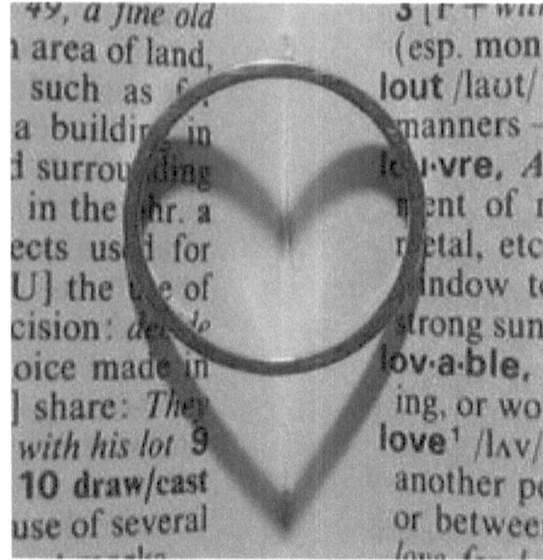

"You come to love not by finding the perfect person, but by learning to see an imperfect person perfectly." Sam Keen

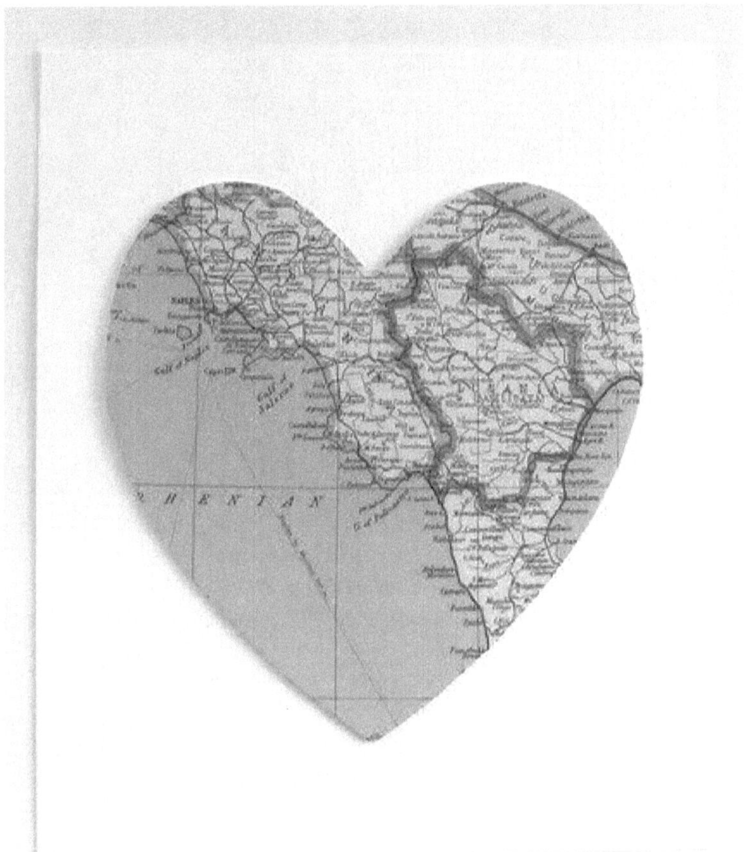

"Too often we underestimate the power of a touch, a smile, a kind word, a listening ear, an honest compliment, or the smallest act of caring, all of which have the potential to turn a life around." Leo Buscaglia

"True love stories never have endings. "Richard Bach

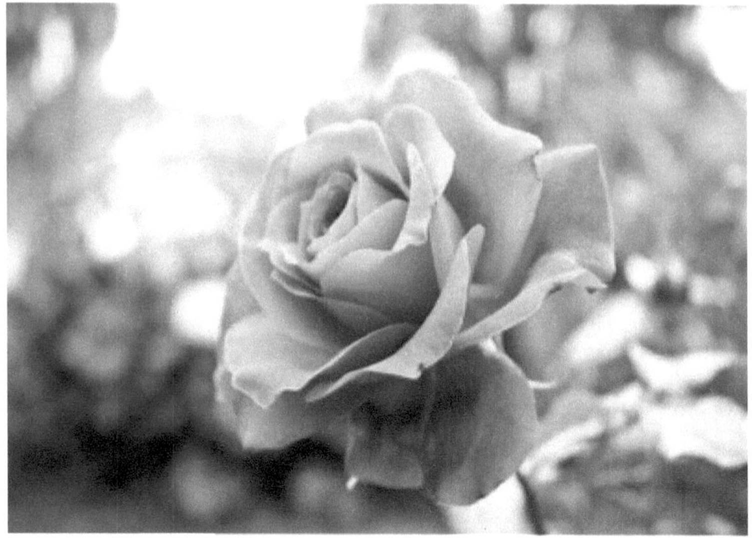

"The heart is the only constant and sure beam to follow ones cosmic door of understanding." Mentor, Agartha

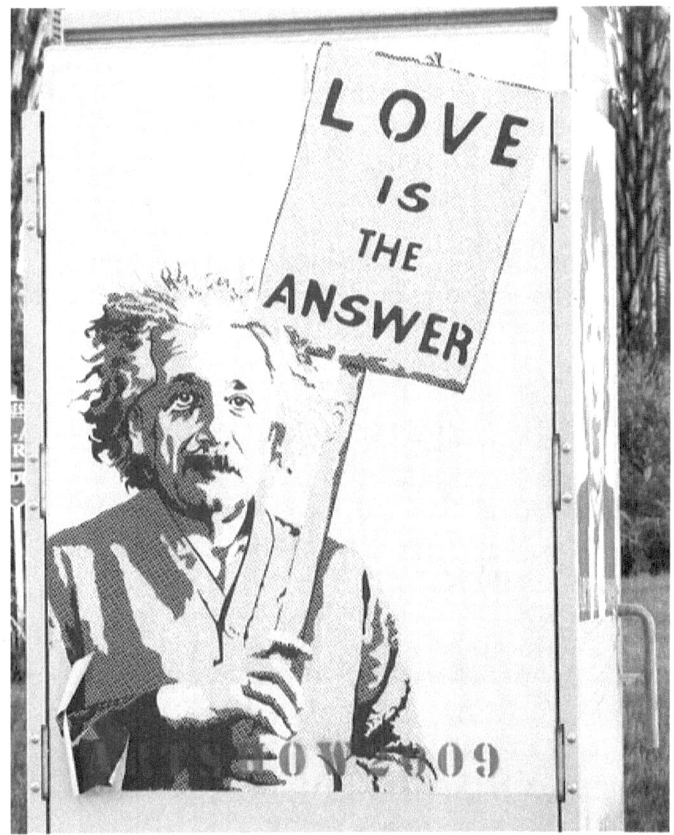

JM

Chapter 7: Unconditional LOVE

Part of Unconditional Love is learning to love yourself—not in an egoic sense, but in terms of loving who you are, your qualities, your good points and your faults—total acceptance of who you are.

Unconditional LOVE… Surrounding you and your being… Surrounding Every-Thing around you. This love is including physically, spiritually, emotionally, and mentally.

THIS IS YOUR **LIFE.**
DO WHAT YOU LOVE, AND DO IT OFTEN.
IF YOU DON'T LIKE SOMETHING, CHANGE IT.
IF YOU DON'T LIKE YOUR JOB, QUIT.
IF YOU DON'T HAVE ENOUGH TIME, STOP WATCHING TV.
IF YOU ARE LOOKING FOR THE LOVE OF YOUR LIFE, STOP; THEY WILL BE WAITING FOR YOU WHEN YOU START DOING THINGS YOU LOVE.
STOP OVER ANALYZING, ALL EMOTIONS ARE BEAUTIFUL.
LIFE IS SIMPLE. WHEN YOU EAT, APPRECIATE EVERY LAST BITE.
OPEN YOUR MIND, ARMS, AND HEART TO NEW THINGS AND PEOPLE, WE ARE UNITED IN OUR DIFFERENCES.
ASK THE NEXT PERSON YOU SEE WHAT THEIR PASSION IS, AND SHARE YOUR INSPIRING DREAM WITH THEM.
TRAVEL OFTEN; GETTING LOST WILL HELP YOU FIND YOURSELF.
SOME OPPORTUNITIES ONLY COME ONCE, SEIZE THEM.
LIFE IS ABOUT THE PEOPLE YOU MEET, AND THE THINGS YOU CREATE WITH THEM SO GO OUT AND START CREATING.
LIFE IS SHORT. LIVE YOUR DREAM, AND WEAR YOUR PASSION.

"The only way love can last a lifetime is if it's unconditional. The truth is this: love is not determined by the one being loved but rather by the one choosing to love."

This beautiful quote is by Stephen Kendrick and is has an underlying truth to it; we are the ones who get to choose our love. We choose our destiny. Everything around us is our choice and we are capable of being as loving as we want to be!

Spreading the love is important and reflects who we are on the inside and outside. If we are able to have a fine outlook on our life, future, and goals, being able to move forward with each step in grace and positivity, our inward selves are being loved. If you are at a good place in your life, keep it going! Spread it forward. Let the love you shine last a lifetime.

What loving things are you grateful for? Making a daily list of 5 things you are grateful for and reflecting back on it in moments of solitude, meditation, or even when you are down, can be a great form of healing the self.

Today, my list contains the following five:

I am grateful to have fingers to type and express Unconditional LOVE.
I am grateful I have food to eat tonight.
I am grateful for my job.
I am grateful to be at peace with my inner being.
I am grateful to have talked to my dad on the phone today.

What are your five?? Make a list and share with us.. Let's spread the love forward.

"When the power of love is greater than the love of power, the world will know peace"

Love, love, love,

JM

Chapter 8: The Story of Ram Dass

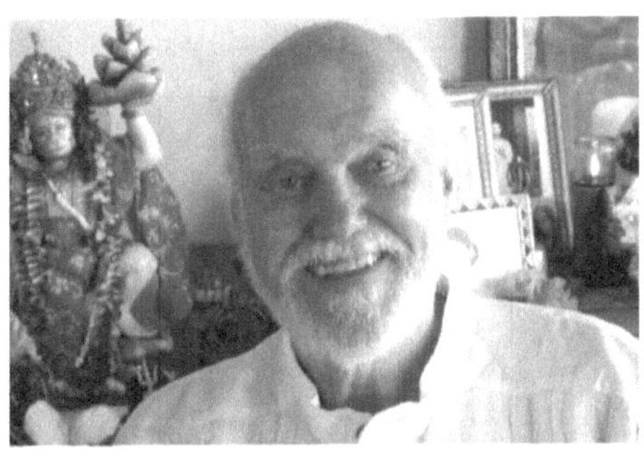

Ram Dass was born as Richard Alpert on April 6, 1931. He is an American contemporary spiritual teacher and the author of the very famous 1971 book *"Be Here Now"*.

I found a lot of quotes from this book on Unconditional Love which are very helpful to a better understanding that state and how to achieve it.

Ram Dass is also known for his personal and professional associations with Timothy Leary at Harvard University in the early 1960s, for his travels to India and his relationship with the Hindu guru Neem Karoli Baba, and for founding the charitable organizations Seva Foundation and Hanuman Foundation.

Ram Dass also wrote several other books including one called:

"Be Love Now-The Path of the Heart" (Das, 2010)

Ram Dass had many things to tell the world about the opening of his heart. His personal experience in how he first started to feel unconditional love from his master is insightful:

Years ago in India I was sitting in the courtyard of the little temple in the Himalayan foothills. Thirty or forty of us were there around my guru, Maharaj-ji. This old man wrapped in a plaid blanket was sitting on a plank bed, and for a brief uncommon interval everyone had fallen silent. It was a meditative quiet, like an open field on a windless day or a deep clear lake without a ripple. I felt waves of love radiating toward me, washing over me like a gentle surf on a tropical shore, immersing me, rocking me, caressing my soul, infinitely accepting and open. I was nearly overcome, on the verge of tears, so grateful and so full of joy it was hard to believe it was happening. I opened my eyes and looked around, and I could feel that everyone else around me was experiencing the same thing. I looked over at my guru. He was just sitting there, looking around, not doing anything. It was just his being, shining like the sun equally on everyone. It wasn't directed at anyone in particular. For him it was nothing special, just his own nature.

Ram Dass went on to become a famous teacher of enlightenment himself and a devotee of the ways of living in the now of love.

Chapter 9: Paths to Unconditional Love

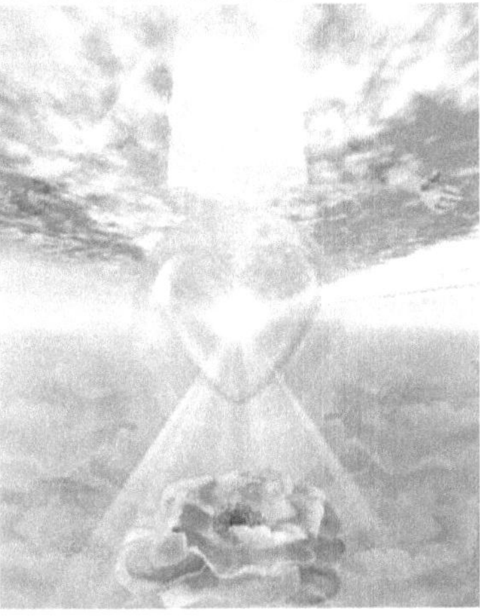

In this Chapter we will look at how unconditional love is described and the ways it can be achieved.

My first experience with feeling a strong presence of unconditional love was the result of practicing the heart rose meditation. (Shown later in this book)

As a result of this exercise my heart chakra opened and I felt this intense love force emanating from me to everyone and everything around me. It was like to most intense feelings of being in love with someone but it was directed outward to everything in my surroundings.

Feelings like this are hard to describe since they are a type of spiritual ecstasy.

The first experience lasted a few hours—a real natural high. Have had that experience a few times since, and learning to feel like that every waking moment is my goal.

Ram Dass (Das, 2010) recounts his first experience with unconditional love here:

> The first time you experience unconditional love as an adult, it may be a gentle melting of a glacier. Or it may be more of a cataclysm, like a giant earthquake that shakes you to your inner core. You are falling in love, but the act of receiving love that intense and all-encompassing changes your conception of yourself. You can't swim in such a vast ocean and remain entirely in the small pond of your limited self. Even if that opening is only for an instant, even if it goes away and is apparently forgotten, that moment of realization, of the heart opening, colors the rest of a lifetime. There's no going back. The lingering taste of that ultimate sweetness remains and won't be denied.

> Dass, Ram; Das, Rameshwar (2010-11-02). Be Love Now: The Path of the Heart (p. 4). Harper Collins, Inc.. Kindle Edition.

What is this state of love then?

> Love is actually a state of being, and a divine state at that, the state to which we all yearn to return. The outer love object stimulates a feeling of love, but the love is inside us. We interpret it as coming from outside us, so we want to possess love, and we reach outside for something that is already inside us.

> Dass, Ram; Das, Rameshwar (2010-11-02). Be Love Now: The Path of the Heart (p. 15). Harper Collins, Inc.. Kindle Edition.

And how does this affect your ego?

> You don't kill your ego; you kill your identification with your ego. As you dissolve into love, your ego fades. You're not thinking about loving; you're just being love, radiating like the sun. That last step requires Grace.

> Dass, Ram; Das, Rameshwar (2010-11-02). Be Love Now: The Path of the Heart (p. 27). Harper Collins, Inc.. Kindle Edition.

What is surrender in this context?

> In the West surrender implies giving up power. But surrendering to a guru or the Beloved doesn't mean giving power to another human being— it's letting go of the stuff that keeps you separate. Each time you surrender, it leads you further in, deeper into yourself. You surrender to that place in yourself that takes you beyond form.

> Dass, Ram; Das, Rameshwar (2010-11-02). Be Love Now: The Path of the Heart (pp. 57-58). Harper Collins, Inc.. Kindle Edition.

What is the goal of this love?

> Although you may devote yourself to an aspect of the Beloved, like the guru or the deity as mother, child, or lover, you are in it for the love, not for the attainment, not for the object. It's one of those wonderful paradoxes you encounter on the path. You can't attain it; you have to become it. In the process subject and object, lover and Beloved, become one. You lose yourself and gain your Self.

To go from the experiencer to the merger with the One requires grace. Know that when you learn to lose yourself, you will reach the beloved. There is no other secret to be learned, and more than this is not known to me. —Ansari of Herat10

Dass, Ram; Das, Rameshwar (2010-11-02). Be Love Now: The Path of the Heart (p. 61). Harper Collins, Inc.. Kindle Edition.

Although you may devote yourself to an aspect of the Beloved, like the guru or the deity as mother, child, or lover, you are in it for the love, not for the attainment, not for the object. It's one of those wonderful paradoxes you encounter on the path. You can't attain it; you live it.

Dass, Ram; Das, Rameshwar (2010-11-02). Be Love Now: The Path of the Heart (p. 61). Harper Collins, Inc.. Kindle Edition.

Chapter 10: Exercises in Unconditional Love

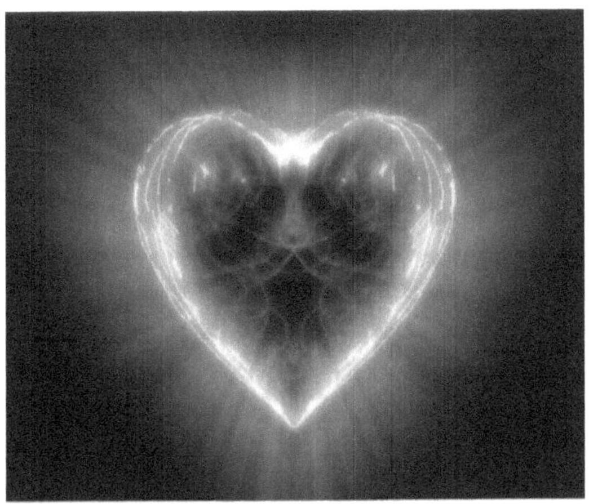

<u>A Loving Kindness Meditation:</u>

This first exercise is a basic meditational exercise designed to improve your happiness and attitude throughout the day and help get you ready for deeper exercises on experiencing unconditional love:

1. Sit on the ground in a comfortable position (lotus position isn't necessary, but is optimal) with your back straight. I've found that sitting on two pillows makes meditation MUCH more comfortable, so try that out if you're finding it too painful.
2. Close your eyes. Relax your entire body. Let go of any unnecessary tension in your muscles, and stop thinking about whatever it is you're thinking about. Allow your mind to drift to wherever it likes for *a minute* or so.
3. Next, focus completely on the inhalation and exhalation of your breath for *1 minute*. This isn't a breath control exercise, so don't attempt to change

your breath in any way. Just observe the natural inflow and outflow of your breath *as it is*.

4. Now, recite in your mind **"May *I* be happy. May *I* be peaceful. May *I* be free from misery, animosity, judgment, and negativity."** Pause between each statement, and *feel* the power of what you've just recited. Absorb yourself in feelings of happiness, peace, and Love. I like to imagine an immense amount of Love energy flowing into my body from my external environment while doing this step of the exercise.

5. Next, recite in your mind, **"May all beings be happy. May all beings be peaceful. May all beings be free from misery, animosity, judgment, and negativity."** Once again, pause between each statement and *feel* the power of what you've just recited. When I do this, I imagine the faces of as many people as I possibly can, and I send each person a powerful intention of Love. I send this intention by imagining my Love as a tremendous wave of energy flowing out of my abdominal area. Repeat this process 3-4 times.

6. Next, recite in your mind, **"May all beings share in my merits, good deeds, compassion, kindness, positive energy, patience, generosity, and Love."** Keep emitting powerful waves of Love energy while reciting this statement in your mind.

7. Finally, recite in your mind, **"May all beings I have hurt in the past forgive me for doing so. May *I* also forgive all beings who have hurt me in the past."** This is my favorite step of the exercise, because I almost always experience an immediate and substantial release of negative energy. I try to pull up the images of the people that I have hurt and who have hurt me, and I imagine us hugging

and getting along with one another. I feel the Loving connection we now share between us.
8. Open your eyes. You're done!

A Shift Into the Heart

The below passage and exercise is from the book "Living from the Heart" which helps one focus consciousness in the heart as a first step towards getting to the experience of unconditional love…

(1) THE SHIFT INTO THE HEART The center of your chest, which is next to your physical heart, is often considered the spiritual center of your Being. For many centuries, it was believed that thinking happened in the heart rather than in the brain. What would it be like to experience the world from this energetic center instead of from the head? What effect would that have on your experience of the world and of yourself?
Exercise: Try this exercise first with your eyes closed and then open. Notice what you are aware of in this moment: the sounds, a thought, the objects around you. Notice if you are looking or listening or sensing from the head, and notice what that is like. Now gently drop your sensing down into your Heart.

This is not a matter of sensing the Heart or feeling what is in your Heart, but feeling your surroundings from the center of your chest. At first, it can be helpful to rest your hand on the center of your chest next to your heart, to help orient yourself to looking from this place. Allow what you are seeing to be seen by your Heart instead of your head. What is it like to sense, listen, and look from your Heart? Pick an object and sense it with your Heart instead of your head. How is that?

Nirmala (2009-02-15). Living from the Heart (Kindle Locations 416-420). Endless Satsang Foundation. Kindle Edition.

Chapter 11: Loving in the Now

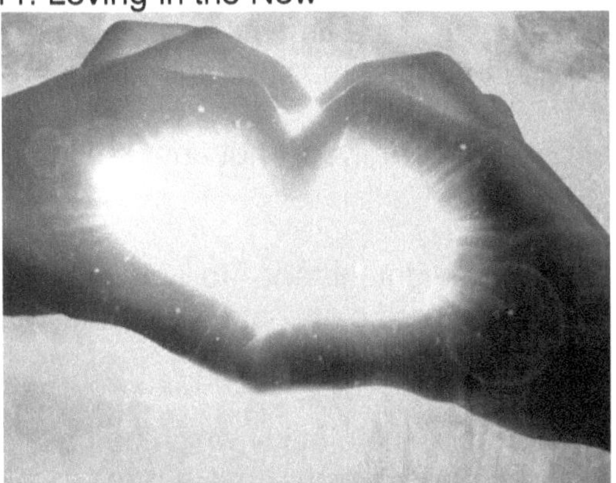

So what do we mean by "Loving in the Now"? (Nirmala)

This is all about the shift in consciousness required to experience unconditional love.
The normal path is to first quiet the mind through meditational and relaxation practices.

Once this cultivated peace of mind becomes a normal part of your life, then you can work on opening your heart chakra through exercises like the Hear Rose Meditation.

It is the opening of the heart and the re-focusing of your presence and consciousness into the heart which helps one to start experiencing the presence of God.

God is the universal energy or force of love, so once we can attune ourselves to that presence we start to feel oneness with God—which is the universal source of unconditional love.

Why is this such a great spiritual state to reach? Because when we do, we live in joy, and the thoughts which might draw us into a "downer" state no longer affect us.

Living in this state all of the time lets us process the daily events of our life through a positive and loving prism.

We think about joy in our lives—not about pain and unhappiness.

This is the goal of enlightenment—to live in the world with all of its attachments and pain—but not let the core of your being be affected.

To live in an unending state of joy which helps all of our relationships and friendships to have a more joyous and positive outcome.

"Living From the Heart" also has some great points about awareness from the heart while living in the now:

> IT IS ALL DIVINE NATURE the experience of looking from the Heart is quite different from looking from the head, but the looking itself is fundamentally the same. To contact your Being, it isn't necessary to look from the Heart or from anywhere in particular. While it's much easier to contact the nature of your Being when you look from the Heart, even when it is flowing less fully, it is still your true nature.
>
> The point of these exercises is to show you the nature of your Being so thoroughly that you can rest as that aware space. Experiencing more fully the limitless nature of your Being is freeing. Discovering that this is always the nature of your Being, no matter what is shaping or limiting your experience of it, is even more freeing. You can rest in this essential awareness no matter what is happening or how you are experiencing it. Just as you don't need to see your car to know it exists, you don't need to have a rich and full experience of your Being in every moment to know it exists. It is always here. It's what is living you.
> This alive awareness and spaciousness is the nature of you. It is your divine nature. You are divine. Even when you are contracted and confused, you are divine. It's all divine. That is all there is, and you are that.
>
> Nirmala (2009-02-15). Living from the Heart (pp. 81-82). Endless Satsang Foundation. Kindle Edition.

Imagine the Greatest Love in Your Life

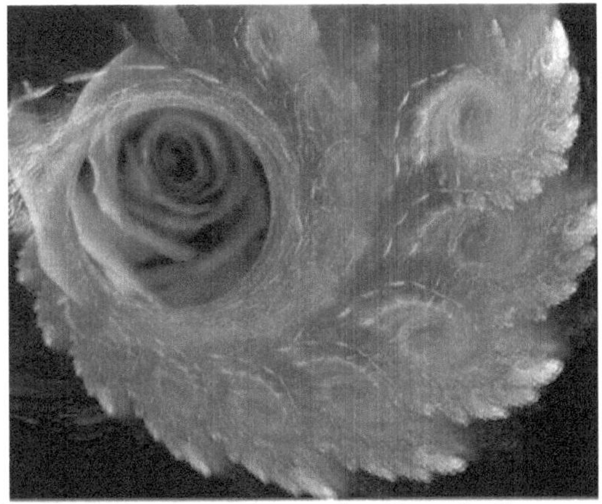

Imagine that you have a close significant other and how you feel about them:
(I'll use my ideal vision of a woman as my subject since I'm a guy)

- She makes me happy to be near her
- Her beauty is stunning and I hold her in awe
- She loves the same things I do including places to go, things to do, and foods to eat
- Not being with her makes me feel empty
- She creates joy in me just being there for me.
- I want to hold her close always
- I want to make love to her
- I want to have children with her
- When we fight there is still a background of love
- I want to spend my life with her
- Thinking about life without her is unimaginable
- Losing her from my life would be like cutting off a limb

- Finding out that she has problems or limitations only make me love her more since it makes her seem more of a real person
- She is the woman of my dreams
- Being with her makes my heart sing
- We both love God and want to reach oneness

Now if you can imagine a person in your life like the above—then imagine those feelings streaming out of you all of the time for everything in the universe—all living things and everything around you.

Now increase these feelings a hundred fold and imagine that this force of love is what is streaming out of you like a brilliant light.

If you can imagine all this—then maybe you can start to glimpse the full state of Unconditional Love resting in the hands of God—except not directed to a single person—but to everyone and everything around you.

Chapter 12: Summary of Love from the Heart

Love is more than an abstraction or strong feeling; it is one of the fundamental reasons for living.

From a spiritual perspective the enlightened masters and even the Bible all say that God is Love. That without this force of love in God there would be no Universe.

What could be a more important subject to write about that this?

I know that nothing I've said here is totally unique—since love has been discussed forever.

I just hope I gave you the reader some new food for thought and helped to lighten your day. ☺

With Love to you all.

Our Illusions

From the Book "Removing Illusions to Find Happiness

Chapter 2: Lack of Happiness is due to illusions

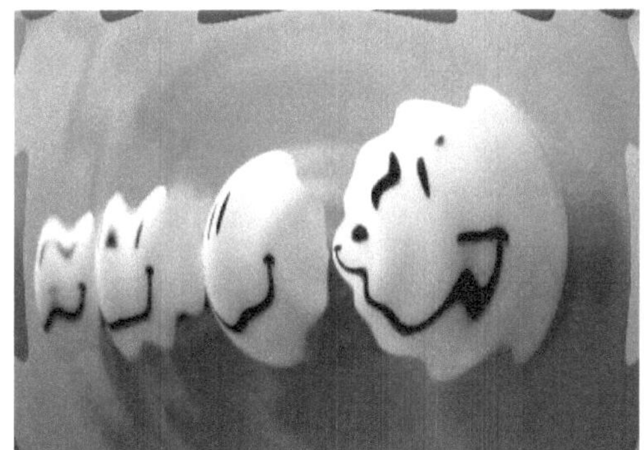

Figure 1-Illustrating the Illusion of Happiness

Fortunes are made selling self-help books. Why? Because, most people are not happy—and they want somebody to tell them the magic formula to become happy.

To be happy you have to be satisfied with the way your life is now and not want to change it. Everyone is looking for something they can learn or read to become happier.

Almost all of us want more than we have and more than our current life offers us.
Great religions, religious teachers, gurus, and self-help teachers all fill the need of people for direction on how to become happy and fulfilled.

I maintain that happiness has a lot to do with the illusions we internalize as "laws" inside ourselves which bound what we allow ourselves to think, to do, and to become.

An example: A man has built a relationship with a woman and asks her to marry him. She says no and the man feels rejected and depressed.

This man may feel bad for several reasons:

- He feels the loss of her attention which normally makes him feel good.
- He feels inadequate to her and this hurts his self image
- The future he was envisioning with her is now gone.

Sadly, all of these perceptions by the man are illusions of the ego and should really be seen as follows:

- The man has a false sense of value in his ego which the woman "strokes" to increase his perceived value.
- His personal value as a man is tied up in her opinion of him rather than his value being based on who he is as an eternal spirit at his core
- His future vision was probably based on an illusion of what would make him happy.

I'm not suggesting that a person should avoid relationships or not marry. What I am saying is that our perceptions of why we want to do many things are illusions of the ego.

A quote from an article I found provides a view into the situation most people exist in which affects their happiness:

> (2) Happiness is a very serious matter and the common human being is very far from real happiness the way one lives and with all the psychological problems inside oneself. Of course,

living in the open sanatorium named Earth, one can only have several fears, a confused mind and a heavy heart. One's life is full of suffering and deceptions...

Depression is so common today that even teenagers are depressed. Their psychological problem is so grave that it has become a neurosis: they cut their bodies when they are sad.

In this world with such a reality, *how can you be happy? Be realistic.*

Only if you transform your psyche and reach wisdom, you will discover internal peace and understand how you can help world peace with your work, in your own neighborhood, family, and everywhere that you play an important role and you have to give your answer as a human being.

Real happiness is a transformation and an obligation.

You'll only feel fine if your world is safe, and your world will change only when the human being becomes totally human, instead of being a wild beast that can only kill and destroy.

In later chapters in this book we will explore the illusions we live within our daily lives and attempt to break those bounds or limits to reach a more satisfying and ultimately healthier state of being.

This exploration starts with trying to define what an illusion is.

Chapter 6: The Ego makes true happiness impossible

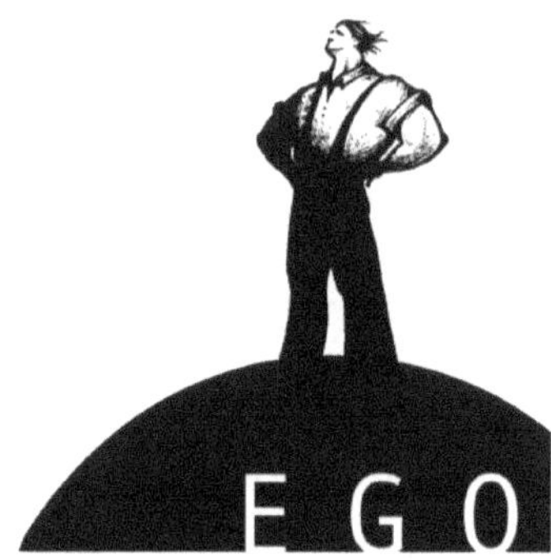

Figure 2-The Ego and its desire for power

When we are born we are pure and without an Ego. I remember my birth and did not have a focused central Ego when I was born. One day on the living room floor when I was two years old I remember saying to myself "I'm alive— I notice things around me." This was my first self-realization of the Ego I had already built.

As we grow, the Ego starts to develop like a shell around our spirit. The Ego is what most of us think of as "I". It wants, it desires, it demands…..and when Ego doesn't get what it wants it becomes angry or depressed.

The Ego is a term commonly heard since it is used by psychologists a lot, but it is often misunderstood by most people.

Also the way psychologists use the word Ego may be different than it is often used in metaphysics and religious discussions and writings.

When I say Ego I mean an actual part of our energy body that builds an energy shell around our spirit. Most of our everyday experiences build this "shell" which becomes more solid and harder to crack or break as we become older.

Most of our culture focuses on the enhancement and satisfaction of this Ego shell.
The problem is that The Ego is not our true self but an illusion of our true self. Therefore, the more we try to satisfy it the more we will become frustrated because the Ego can never be fully satisfied.

This is because the Ego is all about making you feel separate from other people and your surroundings.

Examples are how you feel "better than others", or "Smarter than others" or "Richer than others".

Love becomes an exercise in Ego because it often determines our self-worth such as:

- My girlfriend/boyfriend wants to be with me so I must be better than the other men available.
- Or—I just got a PHD in Physics from M.I.T. so I am smarter than a lot of other people and I will get to work on neat things that will be more fun and which will make me "happier" than I might otherwise be.
- I am in charge of a lot of people at work so I must be smarter and better than them.

The important point to keep in mind is that the Ego is the basis of all illusions, and those illusions are also what create false happiness.

In the next Chapter we discuss more about how the Ego creates illusions.

Chapter 16: Limited Lifespan is an Illusion

Almost all of us have an illusion about how long the human lifespan is and it is re-enforced at every opportunity by society.
We are told we are expected to retire at a certain age, and then get more infirm and sick as we get older, and eventually pass away in our seventies or eighties of "natural causes".
In my book "Immortality: A History and How to Guide" I discuss the misconceptions people have about how long they can live. Also provided are many examples of very long lived persons. (Available on my website at http://mkettingtonbooks.com)
If there were only a few examples of long lived persons the belief in very long lives might be wrong, but there are many records of such persons which are documented in my book.
In the Immortality book I also provide spiritual, energy body and physical exercises and supplements they can use to live to one hundred fifty years or more.
   a.   Long Lived Persons

   Here an excerpt below of one person who lived to 256 years. (There are many more persons listed in the book who lived over 150 years.)

Below is an excerpt of an article from the New York Times (2):
<u>The New York Times, Saturday, May 6, 1933</u>
LI CHING-YUN DEAD; GAVE HIS AGE AS 197
"Keep Quiet heart, Sit Like a Tortoise, Sleep Like a Dog," His advice for a Long Life. Inquiry Put Age At 256.

Reported to have buried 23 wives and had 180 descendants – sold herbs for first 100 years.
Peiping, May 5 – Li Ching-Yun, a resident of Kaihsien, in the Province of Szechwan, who contended that he was one of the world's oldest men and said he was born in 1736 – which would make him 197 years old – died today.

A Chinese dispatch from Chungking telling of Mr. Li's death said he attributed his longevity to peace of mind and that it was his belief every one could live at least a century by attaining inward calm.

Compared with estimates of Li Ching-Yun's age in

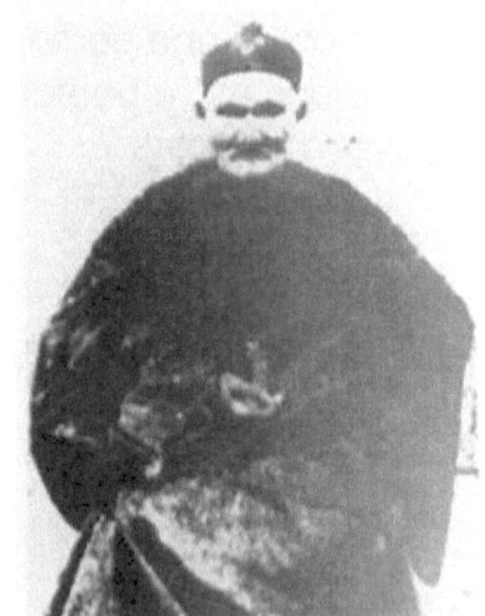

Figure 3-Picture of Li Ching-

previous reports from China the above dispatch is conservative. In 1930 it was said Professor Wu Chung-chien, dean of the department of Education in Minkuo University, had found records showing Li was born in 1677 and that Imperial Chinese Government congratulated him on his 150th and 200th birthdays.

A correspondent of The New York Times wrote in 1928 that many of the oldest men in Li's neighborhood asserted their grandfathers knew him as boys and that he was then a grown man.

According to the generally accepted tales told in his province. Li was able to read and write as a child, and by his tenth birthday had traveled in Kansu, Shansi, Tibet, Annam, Siam and Manchuria gathering herbs. For the first hundred years he continued at this occupation. Then he switched to selling herbs gathered by others.

Wu Pei-fu, the warlord, took Li into his house to learn the secret of living to 250. Another pupil said Li told him to "keep a quiet heart, sit like a tortoise, walk sprightly like a pigeon and sleep like a dog."

According to one version of Li's married life he had buried away twenty-three wives and was living with his twenty-four, a woman of '60.' Another account, which in 1928 credited him with 180 living descendants, comprising eleven generations, recorded only fourteen marriages. This second authority said his eyesight was good; also, that the finger nails of his right hand were very long, and "long" for a Chinese might mean longer than any finger nails ever dreamed of in the United States.

One statement of The Times correspondent which probably caused skeptical readers to believe Li was born more recently that 1677, was that "many who have seen him recently declare that his facial appearance is no different from that of persons two centuries his junior."

After providing examples of long lived persons I also talked about some beliefs that we have a "death wish" in our minds from our childhood. One writer Lenard Orr believed that this illusion about the length of our lives which we internalize causes us to die earlier than we have to.

b. Breaking the Habit of Dying

Leonard Orr was an unconventional thinker of the 1960s and 1970s.

He started the re-birthing movement in San Francisco during the 1960's New Age era in San Francisco. He also wrote a book called "Breaking the Death Habit" which is now out of print.

In this book he says that he met many immortals in India and the Himalayas who were all at least 300 years old or more.

He learned a lot of his knowledge from an ascended master "Babaji" who has been around for thousands of years.

He says that first disciples need to work on developing a philosophy of physical immortality. He says:

"The physiology of physical immortality is based on inner awareness of our Energy Body. One must learn how to clean and balance the Energy Body on a daily basis with earth, air, water, and fire.

Secondly, they need to unravel the "Death Urge" which is built into all family traditions-through the psychology of physical immortality. By this he means the expectation built into almost everyone's subconscious that we will all live an average lifespan then die.

The third step is the mastery of the physical body. This can be accomplished by certain breathing exercises and practices.

The final step is where spiritual purification exercises come in.

From my studies on long lived persons, misconceptions on dying, and therapies to extend our lives, I'm confident that if we quit accepting common knowledge about human life spans we can exceed what is considered "normal" by a huge number of years.

Chapter 17: The Reality Illusion

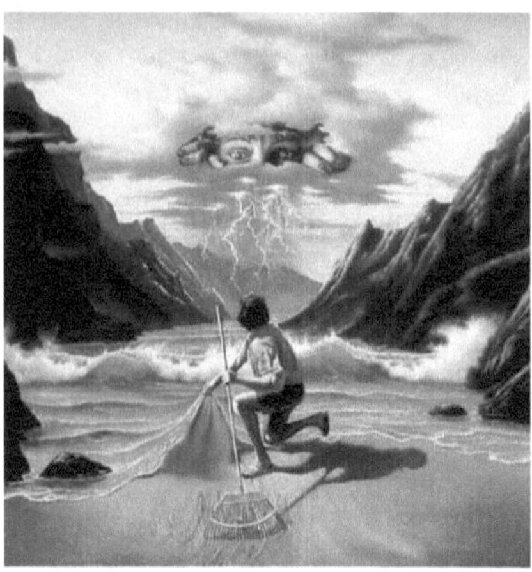

Figure 4-A Picture questioning what is Reality?

Many Sages, Saints, enlightened persons, and books of wisdom claim that the greatest illusion of all is that the reality we perceive is really a dream.

There are many quotes I can refer to on the illusionary nature of reality such as:

- HEAVEN IN EARTH .. CONFINED TO THE DEEP UNCONSCIOUS REALMS ..
  CONSENSUS BELIEF SAYS THAT WHAT YOU SEE AND WHAT YOU FEEL IS YOUR REALITY.-
  Shamballah

- We know that there is not one space and one time only, but that there are as many spaces and times as there are subjects.-Jacob von Uexkull

- You are the entire universe.
  You are in all, and all is in you.

Sun, moon, and stars revolve within you- Swami Muktananda,

- And the Ashtavakra Gita, a highly venerated Indian text, states: The Universe produced phenomenally in me, is pervaded by me…
From me the world is born, in me it exists, in me it dissolves.

a. Metaphysics on Reality

The Yoga Sutras of Patanjali (8) tells us of the illusion of Reality and our illusory perception of it. In fact, this book discusses that by piercing the veils of illusion one can do things which seem superhuman. This is due to a more basic understanding of the universe will allow our consciousness to manipulate it at will.

The Yoga Sutras is one of the most ancient treatises on the structure of Reality and consciousness. Written in Sanskrit, there are numerous translations and expositions on the meaning of its terse verses.
There are also lot of statements regarding the path to enlightenment also producing a mastery by the individual over matter.
In Book Three Sutra 49 (English translation) we have this interesting statement about powers over matter:
Therefrom spring up in the ascetic the powers; to move his body from one place to another with the quickness of thought, to extend the operations of his senses beyond the trammels of place or the obstructions of matter, and to alter any natural object from one form to another.
If one believes in the truth of this ancient book of wisdom then you will see that our solid world is really only as solid as our spiritual perception and belief in the shapes forms within it.

b. Modern Science on Reality
Now even modern Science is chiming in with a related view of reality. Here is an excerpt from a physicist's article:

(6) Bohm (1987) concluded that the implications of nonlocal connections are that objective reality itself is entirely a construct of the human brain. The true nature of reality remains hidden from us. Our brains operate as a holographic frequency analyzer, decoding projections from a more fundamental dimension. _Bohm concludes that even space and time are constructs of the human brain, and they may not exist as we perceive them._

We normally perceive things as existing in the four dimensions of space-time. Holographic theory, however, presumes that there is at least a fifth dimension that represents a more fundamental aspect of reality. Normally, we do not possess the sensory skills to perceive this dimension, and it remains hidden from our awareness.

The holographic model of reality stresses the role of beat frequencies in our construction of reality. Suppose the fifth dimension consists of extremely high frequency energy far outside our range of normal perception. When two or more wave fronts interact, a third frequency is created that consists of the difference in frequencies between the two waves. Since the beat frequency is all we can perceive, we construct reality based on these illusory waves without any awareness of their true source.

A problem with holographic theory is that we have little understanding of why some energy fields appear as stationary matter, while others are manifested as electromagnetic waves. Einstein spent the latter part of his life looking for the unified theory that would link matter, energy, and gravity. How does energy become matter and vice versa?

Bohm (1978) came to the conclusion that the black hole provides an answer. The black hole is an area of collapsed matter where the density and gravity become so great that nothing (not even light) can escape. The escape velocity from a black hole is greater than the speed of light itself. Within the black hole, space and time become distorted and merge into a singularity. While we generally refer to black holes as an astronomical phenomena, there is no reason to believe that these are the only black holes. Stephen Hawking has demonstrated that mini black holes are equally feasible (Milton, 1979).

Suppose that the center of every atom contained a mini black hole. Space and time would merge into a singularity and would become indistinguishable. This would explain how instantaneous travel is possible below Plank's distance. _It may be that the atom itself is a wave form that has collapsed into a mini black hole. The apparent solidity and permanence of matter may be the singularity of the black hole._ Matter itself may be gravitationally trapped light. (Toben, 1975)

So we see from both Science and Metaphysics that the "solid Reality" of our world and Universe is anything but. I had my own experience in the illusion of reality at about age twenty.

I was leading a weekly meditation group during one summer in college. That particular day in the meditation I was trying to get myself and others to get to as high a vibrational level as possible.

After the course I went to my own room to meditate. After a while, when I opened my eyes, the bed and bedside table seemed to grow transparent like they were empty space.

This experience had a powerful effect on me about the transitory nature of what we call "matter".

All of this book so far has been leading up to the understanding of what stillness is and how to remove illusions.

In the next chapter we will learn about Stillness and what is really involved in removing illusions from our lives.

The Heart Rose Exercise

(Video Transcript)

Hello I want to introduce you to a great meditation called "The Heart Rose Exercise" meditation that helped me with opening my heart chakra and made a big difference in my life.

The purpose of this exercise is to help you find your spiritual heart center and to start the gradual process of opening your spiritual heart center. So we're going to go through some relaxation techniques here and then we're going to go into the heart rose exercise and I hope you'll get a great benefit from it.

So first of all I want you to get comfortable where you're sitting or lying down I want you to close your eyes and then I want you to start relaxing your body-whatever technique you use I'll help you in a little bit with one I know--and then we'll go into the meditation.

So one approach is to start feeling your feet. What's going on with your feet tightening and your left foot and then relaxing. Then doing the same thing in your right foot and then relaxing it. Now traveling up your legs tightening your leg thigh muscles hold it-one-two-three. Let go-travelling further up your body-tightening your abdomen hold it-one-two-three. Let go now-look to the chest. In your chest feel your breathing going in and out. Feel your chest all the muscles in it -all of the organs inside of it. Now tighten your chest up tight one-two-three tight and let go now. The same thing in your arms-start with your left hand and the fist of it tightens-that it is relax. Further up your arm tighten up your arm and relax. Now your right arm feel your fingers in your right hand wiggle. Tighten up your right hand into a fist-keep it tight one-two-three now relax. Now we'll go up to the right arm the forearm and the upper arm tighten it up. Tighten all the muscles one-two-three relax now we're going to travel up the body to the neck.

Feel your neck muscles. I want you to tighten your neck muscles tighten them make them nice and tight. Let go and finally into your head feel all the senses your eyes. Your ears, your mouth, the hair on your head. Feel like you're tightening up all the muscles in your face. Just tighten them up relax now. Your body should be getting more relaxed. You should be getting into more of a meditative attitude. Take a few seconds and I want you to start sinking deeper. Sink deeper into a more meditative state.

Now we're going to go to the heart. I want you to feel that your consciousness is inside your heart. Imagine a flower inside your heart. Suppose you prefer a Rose. Imagine that the Rose is not fully blossomed. It is still a bud. Visualize that Rose-keep visualizing it and thinking about all the petals-and the colors-and the size of it what the Rose looks like. We're going to do that for a couple of minutes. Keep visualizing that Rose inside your heart in more detail until it becomes real. Now we're going to see and feel the flower blossoming petal by petal inside your heart. The Rose is slowly going to open up inside your heart-petal by petal-and as it does you're going to feel more of a glow inside your heart.

Keep visualizing the Rose opening very slowly. Now I want you to start transitioning. Try to feel that there is no heart at all there's only a flower where your heart is. You do not have a heart at all in the flower. The flower has become your heart or your heart has become a flower. Now start to feel like this flower heart feeling is working through your entire body.

Your body is no longer there. From your head to your feet you can feel the fragrance of the Rose. If you look at your feet or feel your feet you immediately experience the fragrance of the Rose. Beautiful smell-we think about your knees. Experience the fragrance of the Rose you feel your hand to experience the fragrance of the Rose everywhere. The rose is replacing parts of your body everywhere there is beauty, fragrance, and purity of the Rose.

That is permanent in your entire body but the scaling flow throughout your body that you're blossoming. The different parts of your body you're becoming flowers. Just as you can concentrate on the tip of your finger or a candle or any other material object you can also concentrate on your heart. You may close your eyes but all the time you're thinking of your heart is a dear friend. When this thinking becomes most intense-when it absorbs your entire attention and you've gone beyond ordinary thinking and entered into concentration.

Think of your heart as a dear friend. Thank your heart for all the things in your life. Give gratitude to your heart for everything that's happened to you. You cannot look physically at your spiritual heart. But you can focus all your attention on it and gradually the power of your concentration enters into the heart. It takes it completely out of the realm of the energy you are now just feeling through your heart. Feeling the love of God-feeling intensity of God's Spirit within you and other things around you. You're connected to every morning everything to reach your spiritual heart. You have to feel you don't have a mind. You cannot have arms-you do not have legs- you only have a heart then you have to feel you do not have a heart.

You are the heart-you are the heart and the heart is the center of your being. The heart is connected to the spirit. Heart is the spirit and you can feel that you are the heart and nothing else. Then easily you'll be able to reach your spiritual heart during meditation. So keep feeling that for a while you are the heart-you are in the spiritual heart-the unconditional love of the spirit. That's what you are feeling-that oneness with everything. Feel the power of that love inside you. And you realize that you'll be able to bring yourself back to this state anytime. That by going through the same relaxation procedure and the same visualization procedure to bring you back to your loving heart. Keep feeling this for a couple notes your heart is like a Blazing Sun and the Sun is the pure radiance of God's love. Leading out into your body and radiating to everyone and everything around you. Now it's time to come back-time to come back to who you are-and your body.

Your heart can still be the blazing star. I can feel you back in your body here. You're back on this earth, and you slowly start coming up-up into broader awareness. Your come awake and remember that as you practice this exercise over and over the feelings will become more powerful. It should actually start to feel like a powerful energy inside of you. So I hope you enjoy this meditation. You can do it longer-this was more of the short version and leave you in God's love until the next one thank you.

Gratitude Now

Foreword

There's a ton of data floating on how to be successful in any endeavor. I'm certain you've heard about the requirement for a clear vision, a conviction, a great understanding of human behavior and the precepts of influence.

If you're similar to me, you've likely got a ton of material about being successful. It's invaluable, and I wouldn't trade my material for the entire world. However what occurs when we feel like we're doing all that junk in the books and tapes, at any rate to the best of our ability, and we're not truly getting where we wish to be? Is it conceivable that there's a missing link in our plan for success?

Gratitude Now

Learn how being thankful for every blessing in life will change your future.

From what I've witnessed, there's a really basic piece that gets left out of plans for success. We become so busy doing that we disregard it. There are likewise a few mental obstacles that get in the way and become a problem. It's an easy idea, but it's not always effortless, for causes we're going to go over in this book. It's likewise among the few matters that my mother taught me about life that worked out to be true!

Something We Need

My mother used to say, "Once you get something, you need to say thank you!" Naturally, there's more to it than that, and my mother was merely half correct, however at any rate she was on the correct course. "Now, hold off a minute," you may say. "I work break my back on my business and trying to be successful in life and I've got the crocked back to prove it! Who or what am I supposed to be stating „Thank you" to, and how come?" We'll progress to the "who" later, but for the "how come" we must look at the sort of universe we live in.

We do not live in an existence of random accident or luck. We live in a world that operates by laws; predictable, repeatable, perceivable laws.

There's a law of gratitude and appreciation, and if you're to get the results you are looking for, it's utterly essential that you ought to abide by this law.

Now, what is this law of gratitude and appreciation and how does it function? It's a practice of the law of cause and effect: The law of gratitude and appreciation is the innate principle that action and response are forever equal and in opposing directions.

Here's what this entails – we understand that everything we place attention and emotional energy on, great or foul, will one of these days come out in our lives. The universe, and our subconscious, doesn't recognize great from foul, and they address fear and exuberance precisely the same. If we're placing energy on it, we're establishing an order for it.

It's crucial, then, to be placing positive energy on what we require, not damaging energy (fright, concern) on what we don't wish for.

Gratitude and appreciation is so crucial as it's a really high energy positive vibe of thought. It's strongly attractive! It ties us with the origin of happenings. You can't use a great deal of power without gratitude and appreciation as its gratitude and appreciation that keeps you tied with power. The creative power inside us makes us into the mental image of that to which we provide our attention. The thankful mind is perpetually fixed upon the most beneficial; consequently it will get the most beneficial. Do you understand what I'm saying? If we're grateful and appreciative about everything, we're centering on what we require. It's a way of making a point that we're placing the greatest possible positive energy on our wants, and keeping energy from the uncertainties and fears that we don't wish for.

This is the reason that almost everybody who teaches about goals takes a firm stand in that you view your goal as already achieved, and that you be grateful and appreciative for it – today! It's a mighty way to be certain you're placing solid energy on the goal – using gratitude and appreciation.

You'd believe with gratitude so crucial that everybody would be witting of it. But what I've observed is that a lot of individuals are in reality pushing aside the success they wish without recognizing it as they're going against this law!

There are five cardinal errors that keep individuals from being grateful and appreciative. They all have to do with mistakes in our thinking and our notions, and these are what we're going to demonstrate to you how to rectify.

We're going to begin by considering the question that Einstein stated was the most crucial one that each

individual has to answer for themselves. Albert Einstein proposed that the answer to this was really crucial:
Is the world friendly to our wants?

It appears a bit strange that a scientist like Albert Einstein would connote that the universe may have a prejudice about whether we succeed or not. All the same, I believe he was requiring us to decide if the universe was configured to make it simple for us, or hard. Put differently, is there plenty to go around? How we resolve this question does make a huge difference! After all, if there's a fixed supply of "things" and lots of individuals need it, then life is hard.

A lot of individuals believe this way. We address it as "scarcity" or "deficiency" thinking. It's difficult to be grateful and appreciative when there's not enough. This notion leads to competitory thinking – the thought that in order to get what you wish, you have to take it away from somebody else.

This is a belief scheme that promotes dread and concern. Most sales training is established on this thought. So are all states of war. How simple is it for anybody to be thankful when they believe that the universe is configured to make matters hard for them? Particularly when their thinking keeps producing situations where they get to be correct about how hard it is.

Let me demonstrate to you how abundant the universe truly is. Both science and spirituality evidence to us that everything is made out of the same master stuff. Science claims it as energy. And so how much is there to make more of whatever we require? A late scientific study of the cosmos added together everything they could find and ascertained that merely about 4% of the available energy was utilized to make the whole universe! There's ninety-six percent left over, or enough for twenty-five more universes! That appears pretty abundant to me.

So let's pick another way of thinking. We may see an abundant supply, instead of scarceness. We may choose to produce our success, instead of contend for a fixed supply.

Once we do this, we stop being a victim of circumstances and we start to reclaim our great power over our lives! Viewing the universe this way is the beginning step in the law of gratitude and appreciation.

Chapter 2: Don't Resist

Synopsis

Not resisting is among the most misinterpreted principles of success, and not exercising it keeps an awful lot of individuals out of gratitude and appreciation. Not resisting is merely accepting the mental attitude that whatever is, just is, and we don't oppose it.

Let It Be

Many of us run through life with a lot of beliefs in our mind about how matters that "are" a particular way "ought to" be some other way. Don't get me wrong, here. I'm not discussing easy stuff, like the cars in the street and it ought to be in the garage. If it is, get up and put it where it should be!

What I'm discussing is commonly the behavior of individuals and circumstances that we can't do anything about. We state to ourselves (and other people), "He should not have caused that!" or "The car should not have crashed here!", or "She should not have addressed me like that!", or "We should have gotten that contract!"
Sound like something you've said? It likely does, we've all done this. There are a few things to observe about this, however. First of all, notice that we're arguing with reality being the way it is! How successful are we likely to be acting that way?

2nd, observe the thoughts that go with this mental attitude. Somebody or something has taken our "junk" (revenue, success, love, regard) and we're victims. This is all founded on "not-enough" believing. How are you going to discover any gratitude and appreciation in a batch of mental poo like that?

So this is where not resisting is so crucial. Bear in mind that not resisting doesn't mean you have to be a wuss for anybody. It only implies that you don't debate with reality. What is, is. Rather than debating, apply one of the universal laws, the law of inverses (or polarity). This law merely says that everything has 2 equal and polar sides.

Each situation that looks foul has an equal measure of good, if you seek it. If you truly comprehend this, it will alter your life dramatically, so consider this carefully! Everything that occurs just "is". Like 2 sides of a coin, it has a side that appears "foul" and it has a side that looks "great". You get to pick. Whatever you call it, it turns into for you.

Here's how you implement not resisting in any state of affairs. 1st, you remind yourself that the universe is friendly to you. There's a virtually innumerable supply of everything you require. There has forever adequate money, clients, time, love, acquaintances, and so forth. So that no state of affairs can leave you without those things for long. You don't absolutely require "that one"; you are able to move on to the following.

Next, you cue yourself that you get to choose what to call the state of affairs – great or foul. You understand the good is there (and, yes, I recognize, it's occasionally hard to see when you're in the midst of it), but you do understand it's there.

In my life the sorriest experiences that I've gone through have without exclusion finally proved to be the biggest gifts. They were my instructors, and each one bore in it the seed of something amazingly great for me. Took me some time to discover it, occasionally, but it was forever there. I've discovered that resistance (calling it foul) step-ups the suffering and draws out the experience. Placing the energy on the "foul" experience only produces more of it! The value of not resisting is that it truly speeds the procedure up and gets you to the great part quicker!

So discover the great in the situation, and be grateful and appreciative for it! This switches the energy to what you wish, and is the 2nd step in the law of gratitude and appreciation.

Chapter 3: Be Satisfied

Synopsis

You are able to discover success precepts anyplace, even in classic rock music! While I learned this not from Jagger, the song title "No Satisfaction" details a crucial lesson about gratitude and appreciation. You see, there's a key difference between happiness and satisfaction. And we wish to get happy, but we don't wish to get satisfied. The difference between those 2 words is a construct that a lot of individuals battle with, initially, as the words are utilized almost interchangeably, at any rate here in the U.S. But it's critical to comprehend the difference.

Satisfaction

Satisfaction means an acceptance of the status quo, being easy with the way matters are. Individuals may be satisfied without being grateful as they've just accepted matters the way they are, even while it's not what they truly want. Happiness, in counterpoint, means a quality of mind, a state of delight and gratitude, for what we get and what we are. It's, by definition, a really positive and magnetic mental energy.

A lot of individuals are satisfied, but unhappy. "I detest this cheesy job, but it's the most I can do, so I'll stick it out till retirement." Whew!

What a miserable way to endure!

Satisfaction with the status quo puts a lid on that want inside you that always wishes to grow, to enlarge, to be more, get more, and feel more. Once we become satisfied, we grind to a halt, quit growing, and begin to rust. The place you wish to be is happy and dissatisfied! Put differently, to be tickled with what you have, joyous and grateful for your achievements and blessings, and at the same time, enthusiastic about your power to do even more.

So in the case above one might better state, "I'm not satisfied with this occupation, as I understand I may do better. I'm happy and grateful that I have it as it's presenting me the chance to earn while I learn, and I'm learning what I need to know to produce the better occupation that I truly wish."

Do you understand the difference? Dissatisfied, but happy and thankful. All advancement in society and in our separate lives, springs from dissatisfaction, the ceaseless quest after a better way. Happiness, on the other hand, is the power to view the present and see it as great. If we choose that our happiness is arriving in the future, then we don't have much to be thankful for today.

We all hear individuals state, "once I acquire the job, the raise, the relationship, the home, the success……then I'll be pleased." Hey, I've got sorry news for you, buddy! Today is the sole time you've got. If you can't be pleased now, you never will. View your life and discover what works.

Center on that and see that you are able to be thankful for it! Everybody has something to be pleased about. We understand that what we center on grows in our life. So what are you centering on? What you have, or what you do not have? Are you existing in the future, or the here and now? When you're grateful for what you already hold, you spread the channel for more to come.

When we're able to exercise living in the here and now and being thankful for what we have right now – approving what we have – we have surmounted the next step in the law of gratitude.

Chapter 4: Forgive

Synopsis

We're doing pretty swell with this law of gratitude and appreciation. We've got the friendly and abundant cosmos, we don't debate what is, we discover the good in everything and we're pleased and grateful right where we are. What more may we potentially need to do? Well, there are a few small things. The following one you may not like. I understand I didn't. It took me a while to comprehend this one. I hope you are able to go through it quicker than I did. It's only a single word………….Forgive.

Forgive

Forgiveness for everybody whomever did anything that you've been carrying a grievance about. The guy who screwed you in that deal. The sister-in-law who never paid off the $50. The teacher that gave you the failing grade that you didn't merit. The ex-spouse who dredged you through the atrocious and expensive split up. Everybody. Anything.

And here's how you are able to tell if you've truly forgiven them:

Can you really wish them well? Are you thankful for them? Sorry, but screwball pretend forgiveness won't do the job. You have to do this wholly. Forgiveness isn't something you do for the other individual; it's something you accomplish for yourself. We know that long-run bitterness has awful physical consequences on your body. It may surface as migraines, or heart attacks, or cancer. Why would you wish to hold on to that?

The beginning step in becoming unhampered by debt is to release everybody from debts to us! This includes the emotional debts we call bitterness. We can't acquire what we aren't willing to give. In a cause and effect creation, each thought we plant returns to us multiplied. Bitterness is an emotional bomb that forever boomerangs back on us, one way or a different.

For this reason, each area of your life where you cannot or will not forgive is an obstruction in the flow of your success. The sole way to unblock it is to be willing to free the individual or situation with gratitude for what they bestowed you. Remember, the cosmos works by law, not by accident. There are no happenstances in the individuals that turn up in our lives. And as the universe is friendly, they don't appear to penalize us, but frequently to teach us.

We may utilize the law of opposites and understand that there's an advantage, a learning, a present, someplace in that experience with that individual. We may discover that gift, if we look, but occasionally we have to have some distance from the events to view it distinctly.

After all, whatsoever they did wasn't about us, anyhow. It was regarding them. Once we get to the point that we may be really grateful for them, when we may truly wish them well, then we have cut the chains of bitterness that tied them to us and we're free to march on.

The final step in forgiving has to do with ourselves. There's no escaping this step, as we can't provide love or support to other people unless we may provide it to ourselves first. We need to be grateful for everything. That entails forgiving ourselves for all the alleged errors and imperfections in our life. We have to be able to love that individual in the mirror.

Once you look in the mirror and detest what you see, you've addictions to survive. If you don't like the chief person in your story, then everything and everybody in it gets to be a nightmare. However if you accept yourself a hundred percent then you trust yourself. And whatsoever you wish to manifest in the cosmos will occur.

I can tell you from my own experience that simply starting the procedure of forgiving and showing gratitude for everybody in your life and your past is an unbelievable present to yourself. And it's the fulfillment of the next step in the law of gratitude and appreciation.

Chapter 5: Give

Synopsis

Everything we've discussed until now has been about our thinking. There's a rationality for that – everything in this creation we see starts with a thought! For a long time I played the game of attempting to alter the final results in my life without altering me or my reasoning.

The only way we may arrive at any true changes is to begin with the thinking role. The error a few individuals make is they cease at that point. However effective change forever turns up in our actions. So how does a grateful individual, one who's worked through the previous steps of the law of gratitude, behave? It's truly easy – they give!

The Final Step

Successful people give revenue, time, support, encouragement, everything. As they're grateful for what they have, they give it to others. As they understand that they live in an abundant, friendly, cause-and-effect existence, they understand that by giving, they make getting possible.

If you truly wish to comprehend the might of giving, you have to view everything you have, not as "junk", but as evidence of a swift current, a river of abundance. Once you give, you're evidencing your confidence in this abundance and your appreciation for it. You're establishing room for more to show up.

By giving gratefully and ceaselessly, you place yourself square in the flow of life and turn into both an inlet and an outlet for the abundant universe to go through. Let me give you a few cases of my own. These exemplify the principle that we frequently get paid back in whatever it is that we give.

In my industry, since I deal in info, I utilize books as giveaways. So what is the final result? Individuals are forever giving us books! One of my wife's colleagues gave us a bunch of books and tapes, over one hundred things. Last month I brought up a specific writer that I was interested in to a few folks here and inside a week was surprised with an entire set of his books! It's difficult for me to give books away quicker than they come in.

A different case - in my seminars I've never let profit keep anybody out who was truly moved to learn. I've done this with no anticipation of return - a few individuals have sooner or later paid me, a few haven't. I don't care; either way I recognize it will return to me. Conceive of my delight when we got to one city where my wife is attending school and I discovered that as a partner I could attend and take part in her speaking class and all the particular events and workshops along with the pupils. That's access to info that the pupils are paying 1000s of dollars in tuition free of charge! Isn't that amazing? We do get repaid in the currency we utilize.

So if you require income, give money. If you require time, give time. If you require books, give books! By carrying out the action of giving, you show your gratitude for what you have, and this finishes the last step in the law of gratitude and appreciation.

Wrapping Up

Now that you've studied the book, are you prepared to put gratitude and appreciation to work for you? If so, this means that you're going to have to do the steps, not place this book away in a file or bury it on your disc drive. Here's a drill for you to do. I advocate that you do it each day for the following month to get these fresh habits in your brain.

Take a piece of paper and fill the paper with things you're grateful for. Make certain you've at least twenty-five – thirty items and that you've a couple of items from each area of your life. Include your monetary resource, wellness, career, relationships, playthings, recreation and anything else you are able to think of.

Stop right here and accomplish this before you advance. How was that? Did you have any trouble mustering up enough items? A brief list means that you've a lot of things in your life that you haven't applied the law of opposites to. These are matters that you do not care for the way they are. Here's part two of this drill. Regardless how many or how few you got on your first list, this drill is configured to show areas where you need to utilize the first steps of the law of gratitude.

Take a different piece of paper and make a different gratitude list, with items from all the regions of your life. However, for this list, begin with things you don't like. View your boss with the foul attitude, your auto that won't start, your eruptive adolescent stepdaughter, your ex, the Internal Revenue Service, the pimple on your nose that won't disappear, the bills that keep arriving.

For instance, utilizing my sample list, you may be grateful that you've a job and an auto, for your new parenting skills, your fresh insights into relationships, and the money you have to pay taxes on, a sound body and the advantages of the merchandise and services made up by the bills. Get the theme?

Whatever it is for you, begin with these sorts of items, discover something to be thankful for and write it down. Fill the paper with these gratitude assertions.

Quit! You can't jump this exercise and advance. Don't read any more till you've finished.

Now, how was that? Did you complete it? You might have felt much resistance to a few of the individuals or conditions on that list. That resistance is making it hard for you to get what you wish in life. View the items that annoyed you and decide which of the first steps needs to be used. Go work on it.

Something else you are able to do is maintain a list of what you give. Each day discover some way to give someone something, to portion out what you have. If there's something you feel you don't have plenty of, give that! Be a positive, courageous, upbeat and enthusiastic giver and observe what occurs!

Now to answer the enquiries of who you're being grateful to, and how come. I believe we pretty well covered the answer of "how come." Gratitude and appreciation, we have demonstrated, is among the mightiest attractors of what we require. As for the "who" to be grateful to, you might already have your own response. As a matter of fact, you don't truly need a "who." But if you'd like a list to pick from: Power, infinite, Supreme Intelligence, Source, Cosmos, Universe, Nature, Father, and, naturally, God. There are a lot of other names you are able to use, too, so choose one that fits you. I can tell you, it doesn't matter what you call it. Simply be grateful and appreciative that we live in a friendly universe!

The Power of Gratitude

Why can't you be more grateful? It's likely at some point you've heard this remark from a parent, grandparent or have even uttered these words to a child yourself. (Or even worse, a partner!) Our need to see gratitude in others is a huge part of us seeing that person also as a loving, caring person.

Having gratitude helps us to enjoy life more. It can break through huge barriers and reduce our stress loads, give us more confidence and help us to meet our goals- no matter how big they may be.

There is now doubt that being grateful goes a long way. It's just how to be grateful in times of stress or when suffering from disappointment or sadness that's difficult.

All you Need to do is Breathe

Often we get caught up in a vicious cycle of if onlys. If only the job came through, then we'd be grateful, if only the kids were better behaved, then we'd say thanks, if only I could lose that extra ten pounds, get that guy to notice me, find a million dollars under my pillow…if only, if only, if only.. The problem with if only is that if and when the if only happens, we often just move onto the next thing we want to get without stopping to say thanks. Or we focus so much on that hopeful if only, we forget to recognize all the other things we have in our lives to be thankful for.

So let's start with the basics…right here, right now. There is so much each of us has to be grateful for. We just often forget to focus on the good bits.

Sit quietly. Take a large breathe into your lungs. Let it fill you up completely. Don't let any of it out. Take a few top up breathes. Feel the sensation if it fill your body. Breathe until you cannot fill yourself anymore.

Now hold it in. Feel the sensation of it feeling all tight inside your body. It may feel slightly uncomfortable. It may feel like you are about to burst.

Then let the air out. Let it rush out, then push the last amount out completely until there is nothing left.

The Give of Being able to Breathe

How did it feel when you were finally allowed to release the air? Good? Like a release? If you are struggling to find anything to be grateful for at all, start with your breath. It gives us oxygen, our chief nutrient for our body. Without it we cannot survive. It reminds us we are alive. And that alone is an outstanding thing to be thankful for. The drive to survive is far stronger than anything else. Your world may be crashing down around you, with creditors calling, relationships failing, and stress overload. But if you have breath, if you are alive, you are at a point where you can overturn all of that and start again. Try the exercise again. Do it several times in a row, taking in slow breaths then releasing it slowly with that pause in the middle. Try it with your eyes closed and let it still you. Have gratitude for your ability to breathe.

And After We Breathe? Then What?

Gratitude can change our lives hugely. But first we need to take a look at where we are right now. In fact we possibly need to do a little navel gazing, and let it all hang out a little. Often we are not honest about what parts of life we don't feel grateful in. We know we're meant to be thankful and we don't want to admit that we're not. It all feels a little naughty. So spend some time taking a little look inside your life over a range of areas. Make a little list. Think about the following and come up with one chief thing you are not thankful for about it (if there is one), and one chief thing you ARE thankful for (if you can).

Perhaps these ideas can help you start your own Gratitude List or Journal …

Your finances

Do you feel you have enough? Do you think it's managed well? DO you feel a lack of money is affecting other areas?

Your work life

Do you enjoy your job? What parts do you like? Where is it taking you? Is there any part of you that is still wanting more from your job? In what way?

Your love life/ social life

Do you feel fulfilled and happy in this area? Do you feel loved and accepted for who you are? Have you got great friends?

Your goals

Do you have goals? DO you have a sense of where you are headed and do you know how to get there? DO you feel your goals are realistic for what you want to do and where you want to be?

Your physical life

Are you comfortable in your body? What parts are working well? What isn't doing so well? Are you filled with energy? Do you enjoy the foods you are eating?

Your home life and possessions?

Do you feel you have enough? Or do you think you need more? Do you like the things you own? Have you got your favorite items that you treasure? What do you really long for? Is there anything? Make a list of the things you struggle to be grateful for, and the things you already are thankful for. Don't worry if the complaints list is a little long. We'll sort that out soon!

How can gratitude get that moany groany list looking a lot lighter?

Well it's all so simple really. When we change the way we think, and start to fill our lives with thankfulness, nothing else is the same. We start to change our lives forever, and they DO get better. The movie and book THE SECRET propelled the magic of gratitude onto center stage with a simple formula of think of it, thank the universe for it, and it happens. While there are a few important steps missing in this (for instance, you really need to act on a few things along the way as well for anything to happen) there is no doubt that the step of being grateful for the now, and for the future does help. So how exactly does it help? Well let's take a look:

It helps us in social engagement

What on earth has happened to our manners lately? Please and thank you go further than ever before, simply because no one else is using them! It's true and fairly sad in many ways. If you are a parent one of the most powerful things you can do is teach your children to use manners. And it's not only the words- it's the voice behind them. Parents often will tell a child to say it like they mean it. We as adults are no different. Use manners, and your world begins to open up socially. People watch us all the time as we engage with others.

Gratitude is a way to showing respect to other people. Think about the last time someone said thank you to you and you knew they meant it. It does something quite magical to your relationship with them. Someone who honors what you've given them or some work you've done. If they thank you for it, the first reaction is often to want to give them more. Because you know that what you give them will be rewarded again- or at least you hope it will be! If we start thanking people around us for doing their job, for being kind, for giving us something when they don't have to, then it makes everything run smoother. People gravitate towards people they think are going to reward them for their actions.

A smile goes a big way too. Smiling is an easy way to say thanks. If it's all you can manage, try a smile on a stranger today. They are likely to pass it right on to someone else. It's a bit of a coarse way of thinking about it, but if you really can't think of any reason you should be grateful for people who are just doing what they are supposed to do, think of it as if you are just greasing the wheels. What that means is think about how easier it gets when you just give people a bit of your thanks. Sure, they may only be doing their job, but it's far better than all those people who aren't quite doing even that right? Thank people for the work they do, for any small kindness that comes your way and see how effective it is.

CASE STUDY

Andrew was going for a sales job. He knew he had the least experience and least qualifications to get the job. In fact he wasn't even sure how he'd got the interview. What he did know was he was very thankful to be given the opportunity.

The interview went well, though it was impressed on him again that everyone else was more experienced for the role. As he left the building, he slipped the receptionist an envelope. Inside was a thank you note for the man who had just interviewed him, thanking him for his time and for the opportunity.

That evening, he got the call to say he'd got the job. His new employee was very clear. It wasn't his qualifications that got him the job. It was the card. If he was able to thank him at this stage, he knew Andrew would be able to build positive relationships with his client which is exactly what he was looking for. Being grateful won him the job.

ASSIGNMENT

Spend the next day thanking the people around you when they do something for you. Don't make it empty words. Instead, focus on what the person is doing and then thank them sincerely (and to an appropriate level. Bursting into tears, and hugging a waitress passionately is probably not required if they bring some free water to your table). See how it makes you feel, and if it makes you more open to gratitude? Try and make it a part of your everyday experience.

It Helps Your Mind

Once we are used to thanking the people around us, it's time to start being grateful for some of the good things working in our lives. This can be difficult to quantify, especially if you are under a fair amount of stress or finding life a bit tough. However there are so many things we have around us we take for granted, and often have no idea of the positive impact those things have on us.

As is true with human nature, there are so many things we don't realize the worth of until we don't have around us. If you have children, you'll be aware of that sense of wanting your child to be asleep just so you can get something without them interrupting you, then when they are asleep, wanting them to wake up so you can hold them, touch them and play with them. Or maybe you just have forgotten what it's like to live in your own place, without having your parents around to check what time you get home, or what it feels like to be able to drive somewhere, or go get a takeaway instead of cook… There are just so many little freedoms we have that we take for granted. Find things to be grateful for.

ASSIGNMENT

Take stock of where you sit right now….

LOOK

Take a look around the room. Can you see things? Acknowledge your ability to see. Be grateful for it. Look at the colors around you, how you can distinguish them from each other. This is something to also be grateful for. Think about the things you own. Are they the only clothes you own- the ones you have on now? Allow yourself to feel gratitude for being clothed. Are you in a place where you are sheltered from the sun or the rain or the wind? Allow yourself to feel gratitude for this. Do you have any money on you at all? Be thankful even if it is merely a few coins. These are all small points of gratitude. This isn't about trying to find large big things to be thankful for, but together a little gratitude over a range of different things starts to add up.

So why bother doing this?

If you make this part of your everyday habits, along with getting dressed, eating, drinking and all those other important tasks then you start to focus on only what is positive and good. Doing this doesn't make the bad parts of our lives magically disappear but it does give us strength to cope with those aspects. If you are generally optimistic by nature, this can be enough to boost your optimism and keep you from stress. If you are naturally pessimistic, then this can help you move out of negative thinking and into something more uplifting.

It's so hard to be happy if we can't find anything to be happy about. But spending time being grateful everyday helps us to naturally become happier. It makes our happy state less up and down and far more stable. This improved state of thinking provides a raft of benefits from increased confidence, to decreased ill health, to increasing our enjoyment levels across the board in a range of different situations.

The key is to do this enough that it slips into our sub consciousness. It's said that around ninety percent of our behavior stems from our subconscious self. How powerful is it then when we begin to act out of gratitude rather than defensiveness or negativity? It also becomes a self-fulfilling prophecy. As we become happier, we naturally gravitate to things, people and situations that make us happier. In doing so, we begin to create a life that is all we desire and more. It's the true power of being filled with gratitude.

What it Does to Your Body

So we've got the people around us feeling a little happier and our minds getting the happy message. But what about our bodies? What does being grateful do to our body? Our cells are constantly changing, renewing and mending themselves. Many doctors recognize the worth in a positive attitude towards health In fact, if we feel good about ourselves we tend to look after our physical selves better. We make better food choices, eat for hunger and not to stave off sad or complicated emotions and we enjoy making our bodies move. A happy body is a healthy body.

Many obesity theorists think that one of the reasons that people in poorer areas are more likely to be obese isn't because they can't afford the right food, but that their misery at having no money, and limited resources impacts their emotions and drives their body to satisfy that need with food. And it's often over processed, sugary, body hating food they crave. If your body isn't what it "should" be right now, or rather, if your body isn't want you want it to be right now, instead of focusing on the flabby bits, the sore bits, the needing to be operated bits, focus on the parts that do work well.

One of the fascinating think about people who suffer from some sort of impairment is their body makes up for it in some other way. For example a blind person often has a highly developed sense of smell or incredible hearing. That is our body's way of being thankful for what does work. It compensates and provides an enhanced talent at the cost of the one the person doesn't have. We all have that ability. While most of us can probably mention many things we DON'T like about our bodies, what can you mention that you do like. Some of the time, we carry on shadows form our families' comments that impact us. They don't need to. If you have a chronic illness, focus on the healthy parts of your body.

Many studies have been done on the power of imagery that involves your healthy body fighting the ill health intruder. Spend time enjoying the healthy parts of your body. If you feel absolutely terrible, and there is nothing you can find to feel good, then go back to that first activity at the beginning of this book and focus on your breath. Even if it is labored. Even if you need to do it slowly, breathe in and out and focus on your breath. Focus on how you are alive with each breath you take in and out. It isn't easy. Our physically feelings can often outweigh everything else. We often neglect how our body feels and then we stop looking after it. It becomes a vicious cycle. But to begin to be grateful for our health can liberate us from ill health.

EXERCISE

Spend five minutes a day focused on what is right with your body. If you have severe body issues, or health issues, consider trying some EFT technique to help break the cycle and give yourself a kick start into positive feelings and gratitude. Remember, no matter where you are or how you are feeling, you can love and accept yourself just as you are today.

What about the Bigger Picture?

For those raised in a home where faith was part of their lifestyle, the concept of thankfulness and gratitude is a big part of their culture. You may have been raised to give thanks before eating, or to say thank you to your god before bedtime. Once of the universal concepts is that we all need to be filled with gratitude in part because it is part of what makes the world go around. On the metaphysical level this is referred to as the law of Gratitude.

This means that the universe, or the essence of life around us reacts to the thankfulness and it creates energy around us that impacts us and the people around us. As we are grateful, the universe responds by giving us what we are grateful for.

This is the basic precept in the Law of Attraction that says the things we focus on are the things we attract more of into our life. The things you hold dear are the things you put your energy behind. The more energy we have around something, the more energy it attracts. It's basic physics. So the things you may be grateful for- your friendships, your work, your health, your loved ones, grow and respond to that gratefulness the more and more grateful you are.

There is a proverb that says "Out of the heart the mouth speaks" Take a look at what you say and do. The person with a lot of gratitude in their heart speaks works of gravitates and attracts people around them that do the same. An army of positive people can't be all that bad!

What About All the Bad Things?

So we've covered all the good bits of our life and we're focusing on them. But what about the bad things that happen? Should we be grateful for them as well? Well yes, if possible being grateful for bad things that happen to us isn't saying that what happened should have happened.

It's not about lying down like a doormat; ready for the next punch life might throw at us. Being grateful about the bad things that happen is more about learning to live with the life you've had, and seeing the good that can spring from anything. If you look at people who are successful, often they have a tale of woe of how they struggled, were hurt, abused or injured. But somehow they rose above that and keep on going. Key to this and to their success was to not see their situation as something that broke them, but as something that made them. Being grateful for hardship.

This doesn't mean that the universe is going to give you more if it. It's more of a letting go. You can have two people in life experience exactly the same turn of unfortunate events and manage it completely differently. The person who uses gratitude that they are still alive, still surviving, still fighting, and has learnt from the lessons life has thrown upon them either at their own hand or at the hand of others is the one who is going to be positively affected by having gratitude in their life.

CASE STUDY

Sarah was in an abusive relationship. She lived in fear for five years, and during this time also suffered from large financial issues, and had a near death experience due to a medical condition. She cites the day she walked away from her relationship as a turning point, but she also looks back at the things that happened during that time and is thankful for those too. "I could see that I allowed a lot of that behavior to happen around me and I had to learn from it. I look at life now completely differently from all of that time.

For a start, every day is a gift. It's not something to take for granted" Neitchse said "What doesn't kill us only makes us stronger" While that is often true, it only works if you choose the path of love and forgiveness. Being able to forgive someone for any wrongs done to you isn't so much about whether what they did was right or wrong, or even if they ever appreciate that you've forgiven them.

Forgiveness is about what happens to your own heart during the process. As you forgive for the horrible parts of your life forgiving a person, an object, a situation, the universe, yourself, you let go of the negative power that has over you and you can start to be thankful for the person you are now from that experience or event. It can be tempting to live in the life of what could have been. However this just leads to a stronger sense of loss and hurt and it's very difficult to move on from. If instead you focus on how it's shaped you, and given you a different perspective others may never get to see, then you start to take on a more positive slant. When bad things happen to us we all need recovery time.

We need to look after ourselves and be gentle on our tender parts. But we can also look at the scars we carry and see them as little reminders of how we have survived. Battle worn some of us may be, but how awesome to have made it through to the other side.

It's like Weight Training

If it just sounds too weird to relate to, think about what our body needs to do to become stronger and more resilient. If you want to build muscles, any form of resistance helps. The heavier the weight, the harder your muscles have to work to build up. We use weights to fight against your muscles, to grow them. The muscles actually tear a little as we work them; stretch and then re build, connecting more fibres.

The muscle growth doesn't happen during the session, but afterwards when we rest up and let our muscles mend. To build muscles best you need to work them so they tear a little, feed them to give them the power they need and rest them up. The resting and feeding is just as important as the work out.

So how does this compute with gratitude? Well if you want to make the most of any traumatic situation, where you've felt your heart and mind tear a little, (or worse) then you rest up from it, and you allow it to heal and you add in some gratitude that you made it through it. This is how we become stronger. Being grateful that you've made it through doesn't mean that you are giving that experience power or importance.

In fact it's giving the power to yourself because you are saying that you beat it. It didn't beat you. And that feels good. Learning from our experiences, and our past unwise decisions is about being grateful that you don't need to repeat the lesson again. You learn to read situations that others may miss, you can see things as they are, not as people try to portray them, and you change the way you see the world.

If you are reading this, and you've recently gone through something awful, then this may be the very last thing you want to hear. Everyone needs a bit of wound licking time. But it's something that is good to keep in mind. This is about not letting our life's experiences control us in a negative manner. It's about finding a reason somewhere in all the horribleness to find a gem of gratefulness and let go of the pain.

Sometimes we just can't see the bigger picture

When we are in the midst of trials and horrible experiences we often feel "What on earth that is good come from this situation." It feels like a hopeless case.

We wonder why we've got the feelings we do, know the people we spend time with, why doors aren't opening. It's often only with the benefit of hindsight, when we can look back and see how those times were the very ones that shaped us that we can see it was all worth it in the end. Often the very things we long for and want are not in the shape we expect.

TO get to those things we often have to go on a journey that we don't expect and experience things we weren't prepared for.

CASE STUDY

Rosie wanted to be a writer. She did pretty well in school, and had a flair for words but nothing ever opened up. She too some time away from writing and focused on another career. Though a series of unplanned events she experienced a great deal of heart break and worry that changed her perspective on many things.

Once again she began to write, and people commented don her ability to connect with others through her writing. It felt real, and something others could relate to. Rosie discovered the pain she had experienced actually gave her in some ways the opportunity to be the person she had always dreamed of being.

To make us ready for the big dreams in our heart sometimes we get put into places and situations that build our mind and heart muscles. It might be loss, hardship, pain, death of a loved one. All to build us into the person we need to be to reach our dreams. Look at it this way. Imagine your dream is to own a mansion by the beach. If you don't have the character you need to won it, it won't be a lasting pleasure. You'll let it run down, or worse, you'll lose it. But if you are able to let like create the character in you that means you could look after it, well that would be worth it right?

Sometimes our hearts need to tear a little, build a little muscle and then get a little stronger to reach our goals. If you learn the lesson fast, there is no reason for the bad even to repeats itself. While we never stop learning, and never stop experiencing life, as we learn from each one, the less difficult it is to learn from the next lesson. It's a bit like those muscles- the more you use them, the more second nature it is to keep on building them and using them every day. The heart that is torn then built stronger finds it easier to be grateful, and tends to attract more and more experiences to be easily grateful for.

So What You be Grateful For?

Generating a list of everything we are thankful for can really help on those slightly cloudy 9or downright stormy) days when it's hard to conjure up a pile of thankfulness. Like anything, gratitude is a learned behavior. It's something we find easier the more and more we practice. If you can't find some things to be thankful about, work your way through this list and use it to make your own.

Things You Own You can feel gratitude for ...

* Having shelter. I have a home to live in, a bed to sleep in and a place to put my things

* Having something to wear. I have something to keep me warm when the wind blows, and clothes I can wear on hot days. I can be covered and I have more than one outfit to choose from.

* I have shoes for my feet. I can cover them to protect them from sharp objects and to support my feet as I walk.

* Having the means to travel. I can use my car to get to places (or scooter, bike,) I have public transport available. I live in an age where it's easy to find a way to get somewhere fast if I need it. * I have a computer to work on, play on and communicate with. Even if I have to borrow the use of one, I can use tools on it to find out information I can use.

Your Liberty I am thankful for:

* The fact I am alive.
* The chance to drink water from a tap and it's safe.
* The food I can choose to eat to fuel my body
* Being free, and imprisoned.
* Having the skills needed to read and to write.
* The opportunity to learn something new and life changing.

My Social Networks I am thankful for:

* Myself. I'm who I am, and I accept myself.
* My loved ones. The special people in my life I've chosen to spend my life with, or give birth to.
* The people who gave birth to me and the people who raised me.
* My friends and colleagues.
* My pets, for all their cuddles and our uncomplicated relationships.

My Successes I am thankful for:

* My innate talents.
* The skills I've learnt
* My ability to make friends
* My job, or the way I support myself
* My interests, and the things I enjoy to do recreationally.
* My emotions.
*My choice to love others, and share my life with them.

Significant Moments I am thankful for:

* Milestones in my life. Learning how to walk, to talk, to run, to laugh
* My special days such as birthdays and anniversaries
* Memories. Times spent with loved ones.
* Holidays and time spent away from work
* Being about to order a take-out coffee, or having a meal out.
* Unexpected and pleasant surprises.

Life's Little Treasures I am thankful for:

* Being able to feel the sun/wind/rain on my face.
* Going to the beach, or climbing a hill and looking out
* Washing drying on a windy day
* Seeing a stranger smile at you
* Watching snow fall
* Taking my dog for a walk
* Playing on playground equipment
* Laughing

Things I never expected I am thankful for:

* The things I didn't get right the first time
* The doors that closed to me when I wanted them open

* The lessons I've learnt though my experiences.
Use this list as a starting point and add any specifics you
have. It's a good idea to pop the list on the fridge, or
somewhere you can see it to remind yourself to be thankful
throughout the day. Soon it will be second nature and
you'll start to attract more good things to be thankful for.

Summary

Hope you enjoyed this lesson on having an open heart. These powerful experiences really happened to me several years ago.

When I was nineteen years old my teacher taught me both meditation and how to open my crown chakra and take in energy. The heart chakra is a much more emotional experience.

The intensity of the heart opening experience is still something I marvel at. It gave me an incredible Unconditional Love connection to others and the world around me.

I encourage you to keep practicing the heart opening or similar exercises and I'm sure you too will have this type of experience eventually.

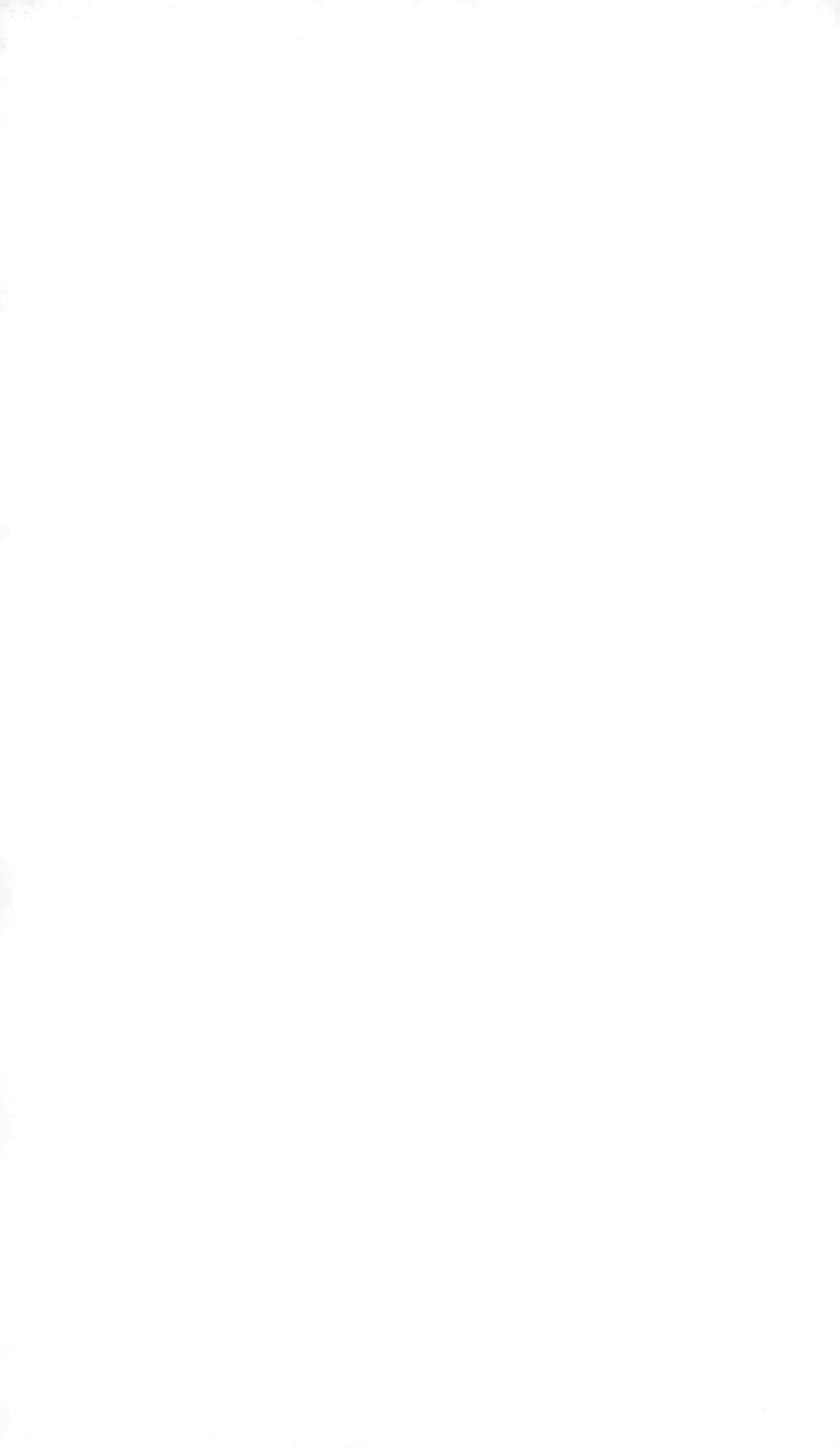